6-8 weeks Baby Check

Training health visitors and practice nurses

Hand book and Training Manual

Dr Rajeev Gupta

MBBS, MD, MRCP, FRCPCH, DCH
Consultant Paediatrician, Barnsley Foundation Hospital
Hon Senior Clinical Lecturer, University of Sheffield
Hon Professor, Sir John Hicks College of Economics and
Management, Leeds

6-8 weeks baby check- Training health visitors and practice nurses

6-8 weeks baby check- Training health visitors and practice nurses by Dr Rajeev Gupta

Includes bibliographical references
Printed in the United Kingdom
ISBN-13: 978-1482654684 [pbk: alk. paper]
ISBN-10: 1482654687
BISACS: Health & Fitness/ Children's health

Learn more information about author at:
www.rajeev.me.uk

Contents

Why we need to do 6-8 weeks baby check 5
What comprise 6-8 weeks baby check 5
What are the advantages in HV doing baby check 7
Emerging role of health visitors and practice nurses 10
Case study... 12
Training module list 14
Overview of modules 15
Neonatal screening 20
Fontanelle... 36
Cephalhaematoma.. 37
Cleft Lip and palate 40
Neonatal jaundice and other disorders.. 46
Dysmorphic features.. 49
Congenital abnormalities 54
Visual Examination in babies and blindness... 59
Congenital Cataract... 65
ABNORMALITIES in vision 67
Presentations of visual impairment... 67
Blocked naso-lacrimal duct.. 71
Squint.. 73
Shaken Baby Syndrome and child protection issues............................. 74
Hearing problems.. 77
Nervous system 83
Floppy infant 83
Meningitis... 86
Developmental assessment... 88
FAILURE to Thrive 90
Heart sounds and murmurs 91
Congenital heart diseases... 96
Breath sounds –normal and abnormal... 99
Bronchiolitis... 102
Examination of abdomen 104
Gastro-oesophageal reflux.. 104
Colic 106
Genitals examination 108
Inguinal hernia 109
Hydrocoele 112
Hypospadias 113
Testicular descent... 114
Undescended testis... 114

Umbilical granuloma 115
Umbilical hernia 116
Examination of hip 117
Developmental dysplasia of hip 119
Eczema 127
Hemangioma 128
Seborrhoeic dermatitis 130
Communication to parents about examination 133
What did you learn? 134
Practical experience sheets 135
Learning Outcomes and Competency Log 136

Why we need to do 6-8 weeks baby check

The NHS Newborn and Infant Physical Examination Programme (NIPE) is part of the updated Child Health Promotion Programme to support the health and well-being of newborn babies and children. The Programme offers parents of newborn babies the opportunity to have their child examined shortly after birth, and again at between 6 to 8 weeks of age. NIPE was established by the UK National Screening Committee to promote improvements and consistency in the newborn and infant physical examinations and its recommendations are obligatory.

6-8 weeks baby check is thus is second most important and vital screening examination for baby's life. The first baby check happens with in first few days of baby birth in hospital or general practice and the purpose of this examination is to pick up emerging problems or those which were not picked up and also to give reassurance to the mother.

There are conditions that are undetected at birth due to physiology of condition i.e. heart defect ventricular septal defect (VSD) becomes clear because the pulmonary blood resistance in high at birth but becomes low at 6 weeks to make the VSD murmur audible, or there is possibility of condition being missed on first examination. 6-8 weeks baby check thus gives opportunity to do a thorough check and also address if mother had concerns about baby based on her observation.

What comprise 6-8 weeks baby check

The first scheduled examination in child health surveillance (CHS) at six-eight weeks forms part of a routine set of examinations which are standard practice, although little evidence exists for their efficacy (David Hall 2003, Helath for all). Recommendation is that it should take place by eight weeks at the latest and should include:
- A physical examination
- A review of development
- An opportunity to give health promotion advice
- An opportunity for the parent to express concerns

The main purpose of the physical examination is to detect:

- Congenital heart disease
- Developmental dysplasia of hip (previously known as congenital dislocation of hip)
- Congenital cataract

- Undescended testes

It should also include:

- A weight check
- Measurement of head circumference (and opportunity to palpate sutures and fontanelles, and assess head shape)
- Assessment of tone
- Check of spine, genitals, femoral pulse, hernias and palate
- Observation for and exclusion of jaundice, organomegaly and dysmorphic features

6-8 weeks baby check is a skilled examination and need to be done by a qualified professional trained in this specific job. NIPE states that 'examinations should be performed by a suitably trained and competent healthcare professional who has appropriate levels of ongoing clinical experience'.

In general, baby checks are usually done by a GP who has a particular interest in child development. In some areas it is performed by a community paediatrician or health visitor.

It is a sophisticated skill that can be learned through a dedicated and thorough training. With practice the health visitor or the practice nurse can perform a meticulous and comprehensive baby check.

In the new NHS there is constant reshaping of the services and optimisation of resources and delivery of services. The traditional delivery of 6-8 weeks baby check by GP or paediatrician is thus in question. Can some other professional deliver this with similar degree of efficacy? Health visitors and practice nurses are good option to provide excellent service. There are some factors in favour of health visitors up skilling to do it.........

➤ Health visitors need new challenge
➤ GPs opting out in new contract
➤ Mothers more open for expressing concerns to HV
➤ HV role is redefining

What skills a health visitor doing 6-8 weeks baby check needs- The health visitor doing baby check need very good interpersonal skills, an empathetic understanding for the parents and other family members, an interest in new-born babies, interest in understanding of the physiological and clinical conditions of 6-8 weeks babies, ability to undergo competence assessment, ability to liaise and work effectively with GP, midwife and Paediatrician.

What are the advantages in HV doing baby check

The health visitors have more rapport and are trusted by parents. Further advantage is that health visitors see parents and families in a variety of settings, including their homes, clinics, GP surgeries, Sure Start children's centres etc and hence they can offer doing baby checks in these settings and thus capturing all in time.

They also spend a lot of time working with other agencies and healthcare professionals who share a common commitment to children's development i.e. GPs, allied health professionals, voluntary agencies, paediatricians etc. This gives them enhanced ability and support for quality care.

When your heart decides on a destination and believes that it is achievable, your mind proactively seeks to discover the way- Brad DeHaven

Freedom is only part of the story and half the truth....That is why I recommend that the Statue of Liberty on the east coast be supplanted by a Statue of Responsibility on the west coast.-Victor Frankl

Thinking is the hardest work, that's why so few people engaged in it.
- Henry Ford

So whatever you do, do well
➢ You are responsible for your thoughts
➢ You are responsible for your actions
➢ You are responsible for your habits
➢ You are responsible for your Life

"For lack of training, they lacked knowledge.
For lack of knowledge, they lacked confidence.
For lack of confidence, they lacked victory!"

We are going to help you creating a new destiny for you, a proud position to help many and feel the confidence of being a winner in the game of life. We will give you training in form of knowledge, skills and assurance to help you gliding through the journey of gaining competence and confidence in 6-8 weeks baby check.

Imagine about the mothers appreciating you for doing the baby check and giving them the invaluable advice that you gain from this course.

Your purpose of doing the 6-8 weeks baby check training

You may or may not be convinced in your heart that you will be good at doing these baby checks and picking up abnormalities in babies with confidence.

You may have full support of work colleagues, parents who are your clients and your own family or friends. You might have done something worthwhile in past which looked challenging in the beginning. It is however very individual and it will be useful to look at your own situation and do an honest analysis.

> ### What is your driving force?
> ....
> ....
> ....
> ....
> ....
> ....

> ### What are your constraints?
> ....
> ....
> ....
> ....
> ....
> ....

> ### What can you do to go across these constraints to make it happen?
> ....
> ....
> ....
> ....
> ....
> ....

It may be tricky for health visitors or nurse practitioners to have confidence in doing baby check which has been traditionally done by doctors. You need to remember that it is only a screening and if there is any doubt, you can contact GP or senior health professional for further advice. With practice however, your confidence will build up and you may become expert in identifying abnormalities.

Suggest 3 things you could do to increase your confidence in baby checks

....

....

....

The course is a self-directed learning course with option of having help from medical professional , as needed. There are theory lectures to make the health visitors or practice nurses conversant with the scientific basis of what is done in the baby check . It will include demonstration of systemic examination and various conditions .

This will consist of 16 modules as outlined. Additional ad hoc top up sessions can be arranged to cover the needs of health visitors or practice nurses.

All the health visitors/ practice nurses enrolled for the course are recommended to buy or borrow the latest edition of "Health for All" by David Hall to have a sound knowledge of child health surveillance.

The understanding of the 6-8 week check will be assessed by course work assignment on 10 topics, each around 200 words. (appendix)

The HVs need to do practical work of doing the baby checks. This will be 20 baby checks observation, 10 supported baby checks and 5 independent baby checks. There will be assessment on 5 babies for summative assessment and a feedback will be provided by the supervisor.

Emerging role of health visitors and practice nurses

While there is increasing ability and skill development in health professional and there are nurse consultants doing gastrointestinal endoscopy, the time has come for health visitors to upgrade the roles. I believe there is plenty of scope for the health visitors to contribute in a much more meaningful way. It may look like stretch but we can modify the education of health visitors, adding additional modules for specific training. I believe in next 10 years extended role of the health visitors should become common and there might be production of health visitor consultant who would be expert in preventive health advice, and would be able to guide and support the other health visitors in their role.

Based on my vision and thinking I have drawn a model of extended role of health visitors which has been published in my book on 6-8 weeks baby check for health visitors.

Thinking of the clinical commissioning and saving 60 million budget in NHS, we need to think creatively and get to cost-effective ways of working. Health visitors doing baby checks is a non-brainer in my view. If trained properly and supported by GP and paediatricians, the health visitors can do baby check very effectively. They have good rapport with mothers and are trusted buy them , hence communication will be easy. The skills for the 6-8 weeks baby check are specific and can be acquired by practice. It will not be every health visitor's cup of tea, but will provide pride and opportunity to those who want to do more and be more in their life.

Potential Health visitor roles

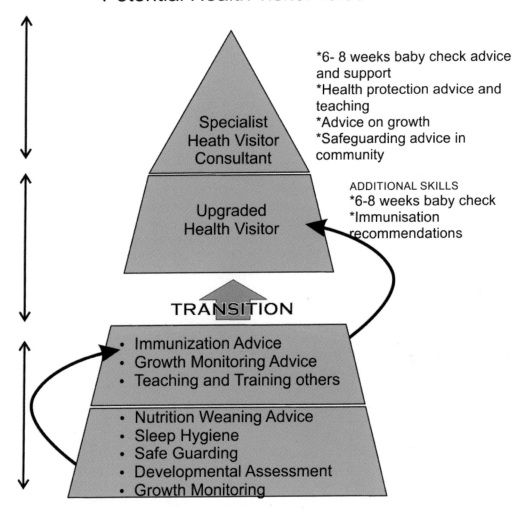

Specialist Heath Visitor Consultant

*6- 8 weeks baby check advice and support
*Health protection advice and teaching
*Advice on growth
*Safeguarding advice in community

Upgraded Health Visitor

ADDITIONAL SKILLS
*6-8 weeks baby check
*Immunisation recommendations

TRANSITION

- Immunization Advice
- Growth Monitoring Advice
- Teaching and Training others

- Nutrition Weaning Advice
- Sleep Hygiene
- Safe Guarding
- Developmental Assessment
- Growth Monitoring

Learning to handle the ophthalmoscope and doing red reflux takes a short time and can be mastered easily. Feeling testis doing a bit of manipulation doesn't take very long. Hip examination needs quite a bit of practice but once understood about clunk, its not a problem. It is important to remember that if there is any doubt, they have opportunity to get it double checked by a doctor. The greatest challenge is heart sounds and murmur. I gave CDs of the heart sound sand murmur to the health visitors that I trained so that they can listen to it while driving and at home. Once the ears get tuned to normal and abnormal, they felt confident. Again, the job of health visitor in this situation is not to diagnose the heart condition through different types of murmurs , the job is to identify what is normal and check it as pass, anything that is doubtful or abnormal needs to go through GP of paediatrician (depending on support and availability in the area). The message needs to be carefully given to the parents

11

about double checking the clinical finding. Most parents are happy, as they understand and trust health visitors.

It will save a lot of money, the cost of time of a GP versus health visitor is remarkably different, more importantly it will allow the GPs to see the patients that need medical attention and thus reduce waiting time.

Case study

I was initially approached by service managers to consider doing the 6-8 week baby check training for 2 GP's in the area where I worked as they had opted out of the Child Health Surveillance Programme. I was looking for a new challenge and for managers to recommend me generated a boost in my abilities. After giving it some consideration I did think there were some factors in favour of Health Visitors up-skilling to do this specific check. Indeed I thought my knowledge and skills as a Health Visitor around the health and wellbeing of mother and child including health education and promotion advice could be invaluable at this important and vital screening examination. I had added skills of delivering vaccinations and qualified as an independent nurse prescriber which could be utilised at the same time as the check. I certainly would not be under the time constraints of a GP and felt that this could lend itself to a thorough examination alongside health promotion advice.

The training module emphasised the importance of history taking from the antenatal to the postnatal period. As an experienced nurse I had been comfortable in my patient assessment skills and the principles of undertaking holistic assessments. In fact I prided myself on these skills. So I attended the training course in 2009 delivered by Dr Rajeev Gupta. He explained the object of the 6-8 week review and child health surveillance was to complete a physical examination. OK I thought so far so good. He went on to discuss the main emphasis was to detect abnormalities such as heart disease, Developmental Dysplasia of Hip, cataracts etc. At this point I remember my confidence leaving me and panic setting in. I remember thinking this is not a role for a nurse and what a responsibility!

Despite my thoughts the training was enlightening and I thought if I gain nothing else I had gained a greater understanding of the physiological well being of the infant. Non the less, I wanted to make a positive contribution to my service and felt empowered to progress and accomplish what I had been asked to do and set out to do. Following the training I immediately identified a GP to help me with gaining the competencies and had good support from her to complete these. Essentially, on reflection the fact that I had focussed on gaining the objective straight away whilst enthusiastic in learning a new skill was the main factor for me feeling more confident to undertake the 6-8 week examination.

I have been doing the baby checks now for 3 years. In retrospect there has not really been any adversity from me doing them. I do not profess to expertly know all the medical problems that can emerge within infants. Indeed one of my biggest fears was missing a problem such as a heart murmur, hip dysplasia etc and at first I relied heavily on the GP for support, sometimes to his annoyance. Over time this has lessened but my rule of thumb remains as from the start that if in doubt don't take risks in missing things and ask for conformation from the GP or other professionals. I certainly have to practice by NMC Code of Conduct (2002) in being accountable for my actions. Occasionally I have picked up on some problems missed by other medics. This is by no means about me wallowing in self congratulations but about appreciating the way training and learning new skills can make a positive contribution to the workplace and the profession. I have never had a parent refuse for me to complete the baby check when I inform them that I am a Health Visitor trained in undertaking this check.

I have gained in both confidence and competence over time. That is not to say I have become complacent, indeed at times I feel very lonely and vulnerable being the only Health Visitor in Barnsley doing this and I was considered pulling out of it. Fortunately a discussion with Dr Gupta identified what a skill I had achieved and a difference I was making which renewed my enthusiasm. I identified that I needed to look at support and supervision mechanisms. To conclude I actually feel privileged to be delivering this service and sometimes we have to face our fears in order to gain strength and confidence. The true test of whether another professional other than a GP or paediatrician can deliver this successfully is to examine the experience from the service users themselves and a future plan is to evaluate my effectiveness by asking the   clients.
.

- Tracy Lake, Health Visitor Team Leader SWYFT

Training module list

Module 1 Objective of Child Health Surveillance and 6-8 Week Review

Module 2 History taking and neonatal Screening

Module 3 General appearance

Module 4 Head and face

Module 5 Dysmorphic Features and congenital anomalies

Module 6 Vision

Module 7 Hearing

Module 8 Neurological assessment

Module 9 Developmental Assessments

Module 10 Cardio Vascular System

Module 11 Respiratory system

Module 12 Abdomen

Module 13 Genitalia and hernia

Module 14 Hip examination and Developmental Dislocation of Hip

Module 15 Skin Examination

Module 16 Communication to parents and other professionals

Module 17 – Assessment Quiz

Overview of modules

Module 1 – Objective of Child Health Surveillance and 6-8 Week Review

Around 2 months of age is generally thought to be useful with a smaller but significant yield of abnormalities, Prof David Hall has supported it in Health For All 2003 . At 8 weeks of age the baby should be showing a arrange of behaviours including smiling and visual following ; heart murmurs may be more readily detectable, and testes are more likely to be descended. Measurement of weight and head circumference and full examination are required.   It is also opportunity to vaccinate, and discuss social support to mother, contraception, depression etc.

Physical examination
The main emphasis is to detect
- ➤ heart disease,
- ➤ developmental dysplasia of hip (previously known as CDH)
- ➤ Cataracts
- ➤ undescended testis
- ➤ Also check weight, head circumference, tone, spine, genitals, femoral pulse and palate.
- ➤ Also look for hernias, jaundice, large organs, dysmorphic features.
- ➤ + a review of development .
- ➤ +an opportunity to give health promotion advice.

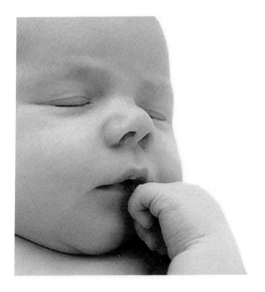

Why 6-8 weeks check

- ➤ You detect anomaly that was not detected at birth
- ➤ You pick up the abnormalities that are becoming apparent due to change in physiology
- ➤ You do screening of whole body (MOT)
- ➤ You ask questions related to possible problems at 8 weeks age
- ➤ You give advice about health promotion to parents
- ➤ Possibly vaccinate for 1st dose at the same time

Rules of thumb
- ■When in doubt……..ask for confirmation by GP
- ■Don't take risk of missing things
- ■Confine to what you are trained in
- ■You will be very good in doing basic examination at 6-8 weeks check

Can you go there?

Basics of 6-8 week Baby check
- ➤ What can you see in 8 week baby
- ➤ General observation
- ➤ General examination
- ➤ Systemic examination
- ➤ Tests

There has been argument about having this check at age earlier than 6 weeks in view of better outcome of developmental dysplasia of hip and jaundice resulting from biliary atresia. However is this is done too early , parents are less likely to attend and opportunity for vaccination is lost. The examination should therefore be completed between 6-8 weeks and if there is any suspicion of problem, they should be referred urgently.

There has been delay in baby check up to 11 weeks in many places due to various reasons and health visitors may in future be great way to offer baby check at home.

Module 2 history taking and Antenatal conditions

Module 3 Screening

- ➤ Routine screening tests,
- ➤ Guthrie screening
- ➤ Common abnormalities expected
- ➤ Interpretation.
- ➤ What to do in case of abnormality?
- ➤ Referral process
- ➤ Assessment case scenario
- ➤ Purpose to determine competence

Module 4 Hearing

- ➤ Common problems associated with hearing
- ➤ Genetic and Non Genetic
- ➤ Questions to ask parents
- ➤ What to look for in examination
- ➤ Referral process

Module 5 Vision

- ➤ The use of the ophthalmoscope
- ➤ How to test for common conditions/common abnormalities
- ➤ Pupilliary reactions/red reflexes/ fixation and following
- ➤ Squint- Types
- ➤ Nystagmus- Causes
            Referral process
- ➤ Blindness- Reasons for blindness
- ➤ How to check for blindness/ vision problems
- ➤ Questions to ask parents

Module 7 Dysmorphic Features and congenital anomalies

- ➤ What are the common dysmorphic features in the 6-8 week old child?
- ➤ Reasons
- ➤ Common Syndromes
- ➤ What is genetic testing/ counselling?

Module 8 Head and face

- ➤ Fontanelles
    - o Common problems- anterior fontanelle
    - o Early close
    - o Late closure
    - o Absence

- o What to do if detected

➤ **The Mouth**
  - o Cleft palate
  - o Abnormalities of the palate tongue and gums
  - o Feeding problems
  - o micrognathia

Module 9 - Cardio Vascular System
  ➤ Anatomy and physiology
  ➤ Heart sounds/Murmur
  ➤ What to listen for?
  ➤ What does it mean?
  ➤ How to identify abnormalities and referral pathway
  ➤ Cyanosis
  ➤ Breathlessness
  ➤ Heart Failure
  ➤ Femoral pulses

Module 10 Hip examination and Developmental Dislocation of Hip
  ➤ Anatomy and physiology
  ➤ Common conditions
  ➤ Questions to ask parents/ family history
  ➤ Examination of the Hip

Module 11 Neurological assessment

  ➤ posture
  ➤ Upper limbs
  ➤ Lower limbs
  ➤ Muscle tone/power
  ➤ Pull to sit
  ➤ Ventral suspension
  ➤ What do these abnormalities mean?
  ➤ Referral pathways.

Module 12 Developmental Assessments
  ➤ Responsiveness and alertness
  ➤ Grades
  ➤ What does it mean?
  ➤ Who to refer to?

Module 13 Genitalia and hernia
  ➤ What's normal and what's not?
  ➤ Lecture on how to detect common abnormalities of male and female genitalia
  ➤ Undescended testes

- ➤ Hernia-
    - o Identification of a hernia
    - o Different types
    - o When to refer and to whom?

Module 14 Skin Examination
- ➤ Common conditions
- ➤ Birth marks
- ➤ Mongolian blue spot
- ➤ Rashes
- ➤ Nappy rash
- ➤ Eczema
- ➤ Meningococcal rash
- ➤ Bruises
- ➤ Child protection Issues

Module 15 Health visitor / GP interface issues

- ➤ Facilitated by GP

Module 16 Communication to parents

- ➤ Breaking bad news

Module 17 – Assessment Quiz

***

Neonatal screening

Ask open question about how baby is doing. The health visitors and practice nurses are usually good at establishing rapport with parents and asking what is bothering them. Ask specifically about feeding, sleeping, breathing, colour changes if any, any hospital contact or visit, social smile, activity etc. It is important to further ask the questions relevant to systems if there is any pointer of suspicion. Ask about any problems in pregnancy and delivery although you expect it would probably been handed over by the midwife or written in the red book.

If you haven't already got enough details, review the mother's pregnancy and delivery records, noting any elements in the history that require specific actions on your part when you perform the examination and plan for follow-up (i.e. hepatitis, intrauterine infections or drug abuse etc). Specifically, you should ask about the presence of hip dysplasia in the close family (particularly 1st degree relatives). If the family history is positive for congenital hip dysplasia, they might have been plugged into system for hip checking. You however need to be extra cautious for clinical hip examination. This reduces the incidence of missed diagnoses. Any history of hyperthyroidism (treated or not) in the mother should elicit testing and follow-up for thyroid function in the baby. Review the infant's birth record for information on delivery route and technique, Apgar scores, measures (weight, length, head circumference), and any interventions which may have occurred after delivery (stimulation, resuscitation).
....
......

Lot of problems are picked up in screening tests and it is useful to have an idea about these.

Criteria for screening
➢ Clinically and biochemically well-defined disorder
➢ Known incidence in populations relevant to the UK
➢ Disorder associated with significant morbidity or mortality
➢ Effective treatment available
➢ Period before onset during which intervention improves outcome
➢ Ethical, safe, simple and robust screening test
➢ Cost-effectiveness of screening

Antenatal testing- This is used to analyse an individual's DNA or chromosomes before they are born. At the moment it cannot detect all inherited disorders. Antenatal testing is also called Prenatal testing. Antenatal testing is offered to couples who may have an increased risk of producing a baby with an inherited disorder. Antenatal testing for Down's syndrome - caused by a faulty chromosome - is offered to all pregnant women.

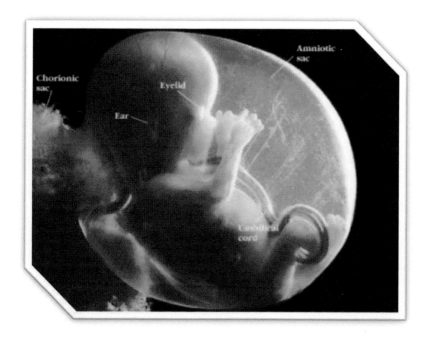

Neonatal testing involves analysing a sample of blood taken by pricking the baby's heel. This is used just after a baby has been born. It is designed to detect genetic disorders that can be treated early. In the UK, all babies are screened for phenylketonuria, congenital hypothyroidism, MCAD (medium chain acyl CoA dehydrogenase deficiency) and cystic fibrosis. Babies born to families at risk of sickle cell disease are tested for this disorder.

Guthrie test
➢ Phenylketonuria (PKU)
➢ Congenital hypothyroidism
➢ Cystic fibrosis
➢ MCAD
➢ Sickle cell disease
➢ Galactosaemia
➢ Other metabolic

Process:
•screening using the dried blood specimen (now known as the Guthrie spot) collected at 5th day, irrespective of feeds and blood transfusion
•Programs across the nation but few variations

•Phenylketonuria (PKU) (incidence 1:12,000) , if not picked up on screening - classic symptoms of: eczema, mental retardation, severe behavior symptoms, often seizure. Blood phenylalanine elevated. Treatment is special diet low in phenylalanine available on prescription.

MCAD -medium-chain acyl CoA dehydrogenase (MCAD) deficiency (estimated incidence 1:8000– 1:15,000).
Hypothyroidism
MCAD
•MCAD deficiency is simply and cheaply treatable, preventing possible early death and neurological handicap.

Sickle Cell Disease• High prevalence of sickle HgB in persons of central Africa descent and ethnic groups of Sicily, Italy, Greece, Turkey, Saudi Arabia and India. Sickle hemoglobinapthies lead to high amounts of deoxygenated HgB, deformed erythrocytes, decreased red cell life span, increased blood viscosity and increased risk of vaso-occluson. Treatment: patient/family education, prophylactic penicillin, maintenance of adequate hydration.

Hypothyroidism

Positive Guthrie test – hypothyroidism

On 5th day of baby's life, a few drops of blood is taken from heel on a filter paper called Guthrie card. This blood sample is tested in newborn screening laboratory for many conditions including test for thyroid gland, cystic fibrosis and metabolic conditions. The test picks up high blood levels of hormone called TSH and indicate poor functioning of thyroid gland.

Since it is a screening test, confirmation is done by venous blood sampling for further testing and include measurement of hormones T4 and TSH. This is done to confirm the diagnosis of hypothyroidism. There may be other tests done to check whether your baby has the normal amount of thyroid tissue, where it is located, and how well it makes thyroid hormone etc and includes thyroid scan etc. The paediatrician will assess and monitor the child.

The thyroid is a small, butter-fly shaped gland located in the front of the neck. It makes thyroid hormone, also called thyroxine or "T4". Thyroid hormone plays a vital role in normal growth and development in children. If the thyroid gland has not developed properly, it will not produce enough T4 for normal body growth and brain development. The thyroid is under control of the pituitary, or "master gland," located at the base of the brain. If the amount of T4 in the body is too low, the pituitary senses it and releases a hormone, thyroid-stimulating hormone (TSH). The TSH stimulates the normal thyroid gland to produce more T4. When the thyroid gland produces enough T4 for the body's needs, no extra stimulation is needed, and the TSH level drops to the usual low level. In most hypothyroid babies, the thyroid gland has not developed properly and cannot produce enough T4. Consequently, the pituitary works very hard to stimulate the thyroid gland by producing high levels of TSH. As a result, these babies have a low T4 and a high TSH level.

About one in every 4000 babies is born with hypothyroidism. The likelihood of having another baby with hypothyroidism is only slightly higher than the one in 4000 chance. In the rare inherited forms of hypothyroidism, the chances are greater. There is presently no reliable way of detecting hypothyroidism before birth.

CLINICAL FEATURES: The effects of hypothyroidism are seen in different ways in different babies. The most noticeable effects usually involve:

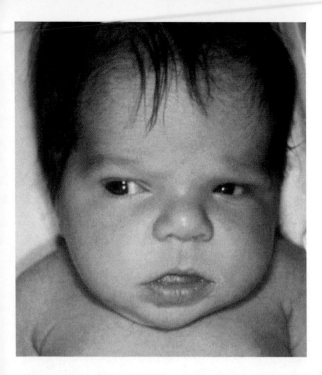

Skin: In some hypothyroid babies, neonatal jaundice may persist longer than usual. The baby's skin may be pale or blotchy, especially when undressed.

Appetite and Digestion: The hypothyroid baby may be uninterested in taking the bottle or breast, and may be difficult to keep awake during feedings. He or she may be severely constipated. Tongue is protruded quite often.

Growth: Hypothyroid babies are often large as newborn infants. If their hypothyroidism is not corrected, they generally have poor growth and poor weight gain after birth.

Circulation: Babies with hypothyroidism may have a slow heart rate and low blood pressure. The hands and feet may be cool to the touch due to poor circulation.

Activity and Development: Babies with hypothyroidism are often quiet and seldom cry. They may seem uninterested in the sights and sounds around them. They may sleep for many hours and often have to be awakened to feed. They may feel "floppy" when they are picked up.

Starting a hypothyroid baby on treatment as soon as possible after birth is aimed at preventing permanent brain damage and mental retardation. The treatment is daily replacement of the missing thyroid hormone with synthetic thyroid hormone tablets (also called sodium levothyroxine or L-thyroxine). The synthetic thyroid hormone acts exactly like the hormone produced by the thyroid gland. When given at the proper dosage, there are no side effects from taking synthetic thyroid hormone.

The dose is titrated by examining child and measuring blood levels of T4 and TSH at regular intervals.

In the lower front of the neck is the thyroid gland, which produces the thyroid hormones. These hormones are essential for growth, development and proper functioning of the brain. The main hormone of the thyroid gland is known as thyroxin, which also goes by the name T4. Congenital hypothyroidism, characterized by an inadequate supply of thyroid hormones, affects one child per 2.500 to 3.000 births.

If untreated, babies with under active thyroids (hypothyroidism) will experience symptoms like constipation, enlarged tongue, swollen eyes, poor growth and dry skin within a few weeks of their birth. The most damaging effect of this disorder is to the brain - it can result in delayed development and mental retardation. Early detection and intervention can ensure normal mental and physical development of the child.

General appearance of baby

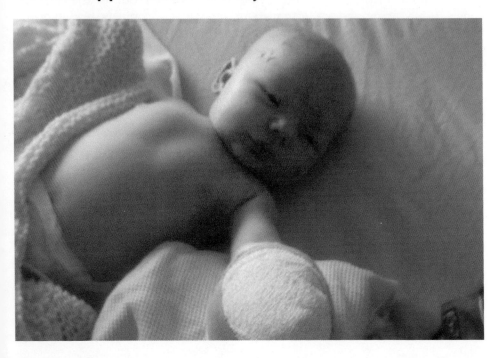

The room needs to be warm, and the light might be subdued, as glaring lights will make the baby close her/his eyes firmly. It is best if the baby has been undressed by the mother , however you can do it without getting baby upset. Observe baby before and while being undressed. It is advisable to count the baby's respiratory rate and observe for any sign of respiratory distress before you disturb her/him (it is also useful to listen to heart before baby gets upset and starts crying).

The following plan works well for your inspection:
External morphology - head size (review head circumference from the record, or measure it later when you start to touch the baby) and shape; number of fingers and toes; proportions/length of extremities; placement of eyes and ears; localization of nipples; any obvious signs of malformation(s).

Muscle tone - healthy babies usually lie with their arms and legs flexed ('flexor preponderance'), infants with decreased tone will often lie with their arms and legs more flat on the mattress, and are sometimes referred to as 'floppy'.

Spontaneous movement - the healthy baby will move her/his arms and legs, and you need to exclude asymmetry of movement. This may occur when infants have suffered birth trauma (fractures, damage to the brachial nervous plexus), and you may find that e.g. one of the arms is not moving, or moving much less than the arm on the other side. Another not unusual observation in this context is a 'drop hand', suggestive of Erb's palsy or lower nervous plexus damage.

Color - the healthy newborn will be pink, but the fingers and toes may occasionally have a cyanotic tinge ('acrocyanosis'), which is normal. However, you need to rule out central cyanosis (bluish discolouration of body and tongue), which could be a sign of congenital heart disease. If you are uncertain about this, ask for assistance or request oxygen saturation monitoring. If the baby is pale, it could indicate anemia/blood loss, and a hemoglobin check may be indicated.

Breathing - Normal respiratory rate for a 6-8 weeks baby is around 40-60, but breathing may be somewhat irregular, so count respiratory rate for at least 20-30 seconds. Observe for flaring of nostrils, inter- or subcostal retractions, and use of auxiliary respiratory muscles. If respiration is judged unremarkable by visual inspections, it is quite unlikely that subsequent auscultation will reveal pathologic findings (though it still must be done).

The important things to pay attention to are:

Face
Head size
Posture
Eye and hand movements
Eye contact
Smile
Symmetry of movements of arms and legs
Symmetry of face and eyes
Fingers
Growth chart
Development

Module 4 Head and face

Baby Checks - Head

General examination
- ➢ Shape
- ➢ Size
- ➢ Face
- ➢ Eyes- Appearance, position,red reflex
- ➢ Ears- shape, position,patency, skin tags
- ➢ Mouth- clefts, jaw, tongue tie
- ➢ Measurements
- ➢ Longest fronto-occipital diameter- head circumference

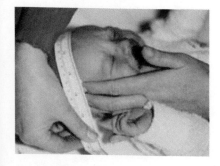

Check head size, shape, and proportions/symmetry as well as Head circumference - (OFC - occipitofrontal circumference). Compare ti to the one measured at birth and see on growth chart if it follows the centile. Place the tape so that it passes the occiput in the rear and the forehead in front, and adjust it so that you get the highest number.

Anterior fontanelle – notice size shape, pressure, trace the edges. Look for any abnormality i.e. large vs small, bulging vs flat vs depressed. Check sagittal suture - trace forwards and backwards from the fontanelle and see for abnormality i.e. wide vs narrow/overriding, open vs fused. Posterior fontanelle - should be smaller than the anterior, and triangular shaped. Check for other sutures - Wide vs narrow/overriding, open vs fused?

Nose - push the tip of the nose in towards the base where the septum and the philtrum join and observe for signs that the nasal septum slips out to either side - it should be seated in a "fork" at the base. If it is dislocated, it can be reduced easily during the first days of life, and thus prevent breathing difficulties and need for plastic surgery later in life.

Mouth - look and feel for any cleft palate, inspect the tongue, gums, and mucous membranes, noting any discoloration, enanthema, or malformations. Natal teeth may be present from birth, and should probably be removed if they are lose (risk of aspiration). A short frenulum ('tongue tie') may need to be cut if only it causes problems with latching on during breast feeding, or if the mother experiences the baby's sucking as painful.

Neck - torticollis (asymmetric/twisted neck), if present at birth, is most commonly due to intrauterine position, though rarely defective segmentation of the cervical vertebrae may be involved. Torticollis may also appear 2-3 weeks after birth, and is then presumed to be due to trauma of a sternocleidomastoid muscle during delivery, causing hemorrhage (sternomastoid haemorrhage also misnomer- sternomastoid tumour) followed by fibrotic repair/organization. Although this mechanism is debated, you should palpate both sternocleidomastoids to rule out such phenomena. The presence of torticollis calls for physiotherapy, and the infant should be evaluated by a physiotherapist before discharge.

Clavicles - may fracture during birth, and you should palpate both clavicles for the presence of swelling or the feeling of crepitation. No therapy is necessary, although paracetamol may be indicated if the infant appears to be in pain. Parents need to know, so they can exercise caution during handling baby.

Head shape

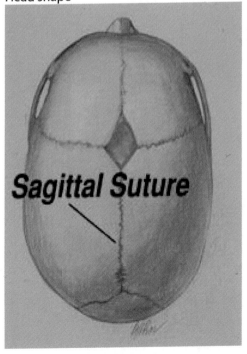

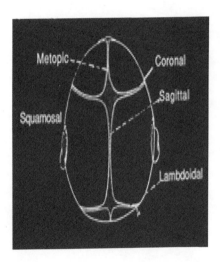

It is common for a newborn baby to have an unusual head shape. This can be caused by the position of the baby in the uterus during pregnancy, or can happen during birth. Baby's head should go back to a normal shape within about 6 weeks after birth. Sometimes a baby's head does not return to a normal shape and the baby may have developed a flattened spot at the back or side of the head. This condition is known as deformational plagiocephaly.

Plagiocephaly - Pronounced: Play-gee-o-kef-a-lee

Plagiocephaly is the most common craniofacial problem today. Deformational plagiocephaly, also known as positional plagiocephaly, means a mis-shapen or uneven (asymmetrical) head shape. Plagiocephaly does not affect the development of a baby's brain, but if not treated it may change their physical appearance by causing uneven growth of their face and head.

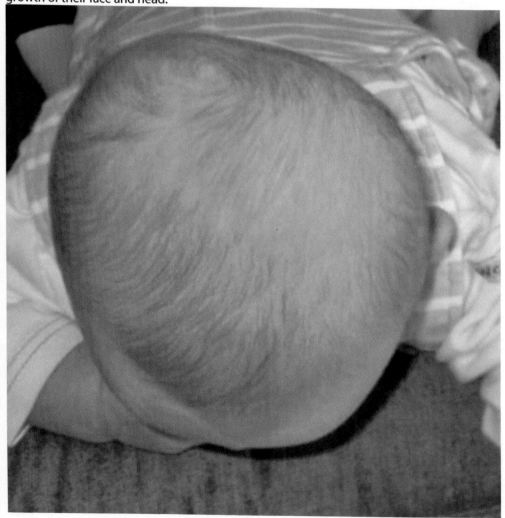

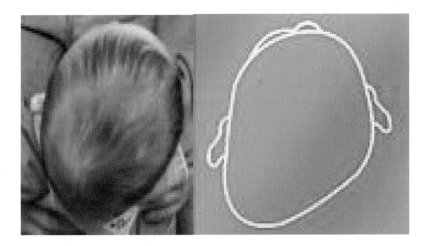

<u>Cause-</u> The bones of a newborn baby's head are thin and flexible so the head is soft and may change shape easily. Flattening of the head in one area may happen if a baby lies with its head in the same position for a long time. Other causes include Prematurity, Congenital torticollis

A baby's head position needs to be varied during sleep and awake periods. There are some simple things you can do to help prevent baby developing deformational plagiocephaly.

Most children with plagiocephaly do not require any investigation or treatment at all. If however it is persist and there is slow head circumference growth, the child need to be referred to paediatrician to check for suture fusion.

•Counter positioning is usually helpful for correction. This involves parents making sure their infant does not rest on the flat spot by alternating their baby's head position from the back to the sides. Increased tummy time and lying your baby on their side to play can also help. Counter positioning techniques can be taught by health professionals. If torticollis, paediatric physiotherapists can help. Some parents ask for Corrective helmets, however they are best advised to contact orthotist or GP. Helmets may cost £2000.

Brachycephaly

Brachycephaly refers to the condition where the head is disproportionately wide. Brachycephaly can result from the premature fusion of the coronal sutures (craniosynostosis) or from external deformation (most commonly prolonged lying on the back -- a positional deformity). The head flattens uniformly, causing a much wider and shorter head. Increased head height is also common in children with brachycephaly. It is commonly seen in Down's Syndrome

Brachycephaly resulting from early closure of the coronal sutures (i.e., craniosynostosis) is also present in many syndromal abnormalities, such as Apert, Crouzon, Pfeiffer, Saethre-Chotzen and Carpenters syndromes.

The initial examination involves questions about gestation, birth, in utero and post-natal positioning (for example, sleeping position). The physical examination includes inspection of the infant's head and may involve palpation of the child's skull for suture ridges and soft spots (the fontanelles). It is important to do head circumference to check head growth. If any doubt about head growth or any other feature, refer to paediatrician who may request x-rays to check sutural fusion.

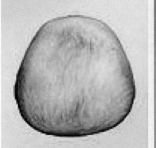 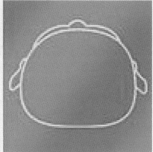

Scaphocephaly

Scaphocephaly, derived from the Greek skaphe, describes a specific variety of a long narrow head that resembles an inverted boat.

Deformational scaphocephaly is quite common and is characterized by a long and narrow head shape, sometimes caused by consistent positioning of the baby on its side. Like brachycephaly, scaphocephaly is a deformity of proportion. Premature babies are particularly prone to this deformity since their skulls are so fragile, and a side-lying position is often used in the Neonatal Intensive Care Unit (NICU) for easy access to monitors and other equipment. Orthotic management focuses on normalizing the proportion and overall shape of the head.
It can also happen when there is a premature fusion of the sagittal suture. The sagittal suture joins together the two parietal bones of skull. Scaphocephaly is the most common of the craniosynostosis conditions and is characterized by a long, narrow head.

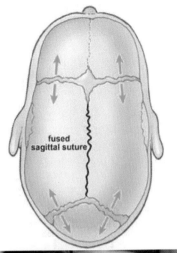

fused
sagittal suture

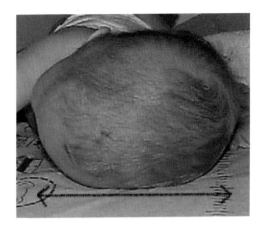

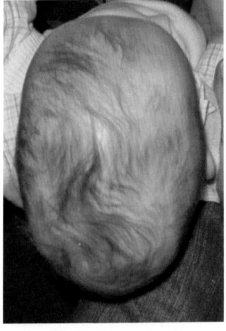

Microcephaly

Microcephaly mean a small head and is usually is the result of abnormal brain development, which can occur in the womb (congenital) or in infancy. Microcephaly may be genetic. Other possible causes may be:

Chromosomal abnormalities. Down syndrome and other conditions may result in microcephaly.

Decreased oxygen to the fetal brain (cerebral anoxia). Certain complications of pregnancy or delivery can impair oxygen delivery to the fetal brain.

Infections of the fetus during pregnancy. These include toxoplasmosis, cytomegalovirus, German measles (rubella), and chickenpox (varicella).

Exposure to drugs, alcohol or certain toxic chemicals in the womb. Any of these put your baby at risk of brain abnormalities.

Craniosynostosis. The premature fusing of the sutures between the bony plates that form an infant's skull keeps the brain from growing. Its not common and need referral to paediatrician for diagnosis usually means infant needs surgery to separate the fused bones. If there are no underlying problems in the brain, this surgery allows the brain adequate space to grow and develop.

.

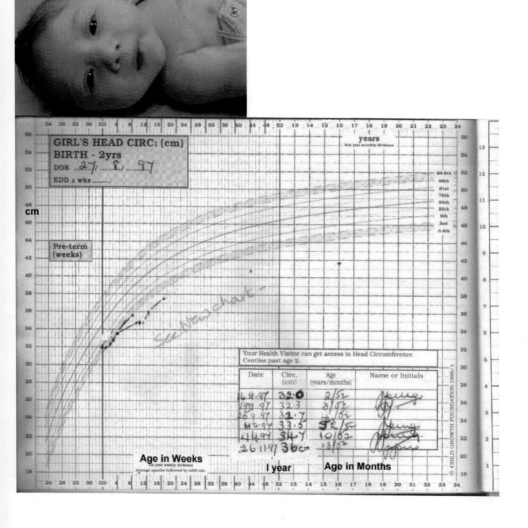

GIRL'S HEAD CIRC: (cm)
BIRTH - 2yrs
DOB 27. 8. 97
EDD ± wks ....

years

Pre-term (weeks)

cm

See New chart -

Your Health Visitor can get access to Head Circumference Centiles past age 2.

Date	Circ. (cm)	Age (years/months)	Name or Initials
6.9.97	32.0	2/52	
19.9.97	32.3	3/52	
26.9.97	32.7	4/52	
10.9.97	33.5	52/52	
14.9.97	34.7	10/52	
26.11.97	36cm	13/52	

Age in Weeks

Age in Months

1 year

© CHILD GROWTH FOUNDATION 1996/1

Hydrocephalus

Hydrocephalus is disgnosed antenatally in most cases if it is present before birth. Ultrasound can show dilated ventricles as in the picture below.

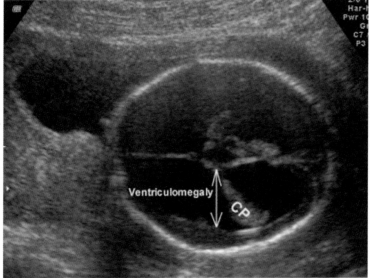

Hydrocephalus can however develop later due to blockage of circulation of cerebrospinal fluid from one of ventricles .

Some of the common symptoms in babies are:
- Head growth that is larger than normal (increasing head circumference)
- Bulging "soft spots" (fontanelles)
- Wide gapbetween sutures of skull bones (splayed sutures)
- Poor feeding
- High-pitched cry
- Sleepiness
- Irritability
- Lack of social smile indicating delayed development

Ultrasound of head is required to see any dilatation of ventricles in head, so a quick referral via GP or in direct discussion with paediatrician is required. The most common treatment for hydrocephalus is surgery to put in a shunt.

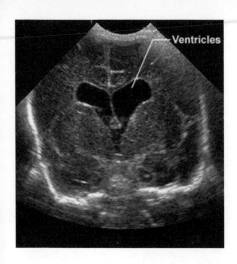

Fontanelle

The anterior fontanelle varies from 1-4cm in any direction. The diamond-shaped junction of the coronal frontal and sagittal sutures; it becomes ossified within 18-24months.

The posterior fontanelle should be less than 1cm and usually closes by 3 months. This triangular fontanel is at the junction of the sagittal and lambdoid sutures; ossified by the end of the 1st year.

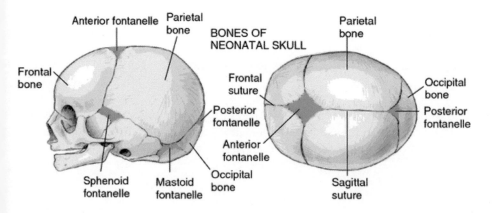

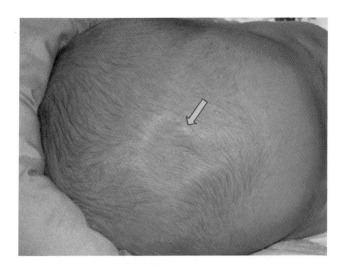

A bony defect along the saggital suture in the parietal bones is a possible fontanelle. It may be a feature of certain syndromes such as Trisomy 21. Large posterior fontanelle may be present in congenital hypothyroidism.

Sutures should be freely mobile. Craniosynostosis is a prematurely fused suture.

Normally, fontanelles are flat. A bulging fontanelle may indicate increased intracranial pressure; a depressed fontanelle may be seen in dehydration. Normally, during crying, the fontanelles bulge.

Cephalhaematoma

Cephalhaematoma is a type of localized swelling involving the scalp and is often seen in newborns. It is due to subperiosteol hemorrhage involving the outer table of one of the cranial bones. Swelling does not extend across a suture (unlike caput succedenaum). It may be small and well localized or may involve the entire bone. Occasionally, bilateral symmetrical swellings occur after difficult deliveries. Although initially soft the swellings develop a raised bony margin within 2-3 days, due to the rapid deposition of calcium at the edges of the elevated periosteum. The entire process usually disappears within a few weeks, but may remain as a residual osteoma that is not resorbed for a year or two. Commonly it is on the parietal bone. There is no discoloration of the overlying scalp, and there may be history of ventuose or instrumental delivery. It may occasionally be complicated by jaundice & anaemia

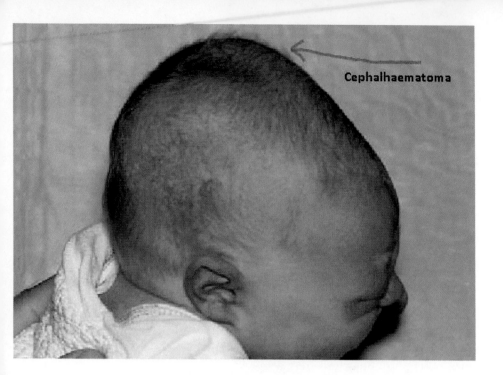

Cephalhaematoma

Caput succedenaum on the other hand a swelling of newborn baby's scalp due oedema and bruising over the occipitoparietal region and should disappear well before 6-8 weeks baby check. It usually subside within the first 24 hours of life.

Faces -Eyes
• Slant of eyes upslant outwards – Down syndrome
•Slant of eyes downslant outwards- Treacher Collin syndrome

• wide –set eyes may be normal or due to syndromes. Just keep a note, on its own does not indicate any problem, hence always try to make sense with what else is there.

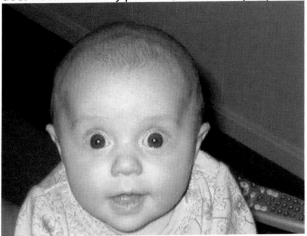

Faces- Ears
•Check for Shape, Low set ears, and patency

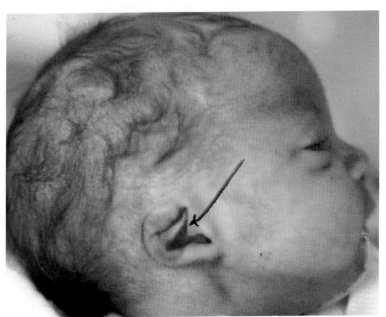

Low set malformed ears are common in many genetic and chromosomal syndromes.

Low set ears, face asymmetry, and heart murmur of pulmonary stenosis indicate Noonan syndrome

Noonan syndrome is a common genetic disorder characterized by facial anomalies, congenital heart defect, short stature, webbed neck, chest deformities and undescended testes. The phenotypic expression of Noonan syndrome is extremely variable, with some affected subjects showing only minor features of the syndrome. Cardiac malformations are also heterogeneous. Pulmonary stenosis, with or without dysplastic pulmonary valve and hypertrophic cardiomyopathy, are the "classic" cardiac defects reported in Noonan syndrome. However, atrial septal defect, atrioventricular septal defect, left-sided obstructive lesions, tetralogy of Fallot and patent ductus arteriosus have also been described.

Mouth

Cleft Lip and palate

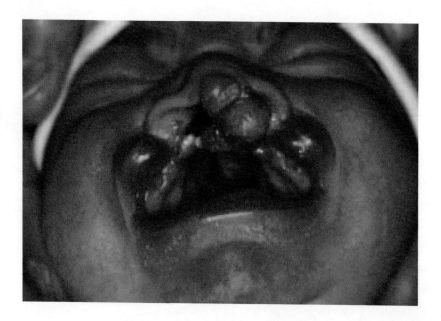

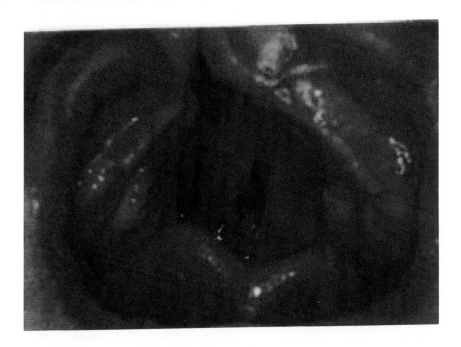

- ➢ Commonest congenital abnormalities of the orofacial structure
- ➢ Cleft lip / palate occurs in 1:600 live births
- ➢ Isolated cleft palate occurs in 1:1000 live births
- ➢ Often occur as isolated deformities
- ➢ Can be associated with other anomalies (e.g. congenital heart disease)
- ➢ Cleft lips and palates are a diverse and variable congenital abnormality
- ➢ Cleft lip / palate predominates in males
- ➢ Isolated cleft palate is more common in female

- **Aetiology**
- ➢ Cleft lip and palate is believed to have both a genetic and environmental component
- ➢ Cleft palate may be inherited as an autosomal dominant condition with variable penetrance
- ➢ Family history in a first-degree relative increases the risk by a factor of 20
- ➢ Environmental factors include:
- ➢ Maternal epilepsy
- ➢ Drugs - steroids, diazepam, phenytoin
- ➢ ? Folic acid deficiency
- ➢ Cleft lip and palate also occurs as part of over 100 syndromes
- ➢ Pierre Robin Syndrome - cleft palate, retrognathia, posteriorly displaced tongue
- ➢ Stickler Syndrome
- ➢ Down's Syndrome
- ➢ Treacher Collins' Syndrome

- **Embryology**

- Cleft lip deformity is established in first 6 weeks of life
- Possibly due to failure of fusion of maxillary and medial nasal processes
- May be due to incomplete mesodermal ingrowth into the processes
- Extent of deficiency determines the extent of the cleft
- Palatal clefts result from failure of fusion of the palatal shelves of the maxillary processes

- **Clinical features**
- Typical distribution of cleft types is :
- Cleft lip alone (15%)
- Cleft lip and palate (45%)
- Isolated cleft palate (40%)
- Cleft lips are more common on the left

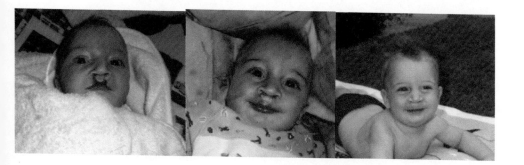

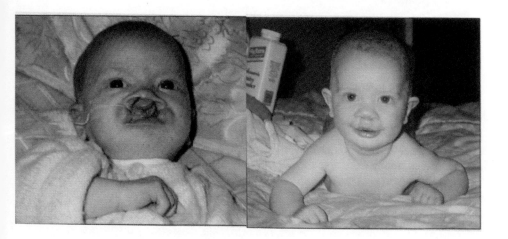

Primary management of cleft lip and palate
- Antenatal diagnosis of cleft lip may be possible
- Feeding is rarely a difficulty

- Breast feeding may be achieved or modified teats for bottle feeding may be required
- Major respiratory obstruction is uncommon
- The aims of surgery are:
- To achieve a normal appearance of the lip, nose and face
- To allow normal facial growth
- To allow normal speech

Secondary management of cleft lip and palate
Surgery
- Many different techniques have been advocated
- Cleft lip repair is usually performed between 3 and 6 months of age ??
- Cleft palate repair is usually performed between 6 and 18 months
- Two or more operations may be required
- A multidisciplinary team approach is essential
- Other aspects that need to be addressed included
- Hearing
- Speech therapy
- Dental
- Orthodontics

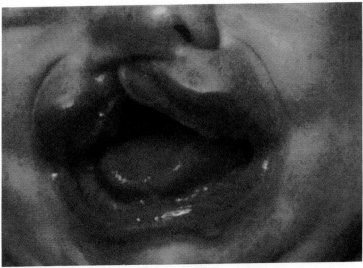

Unilateral cleft palate with tongue tie

These pictures below shows incomplete cleft

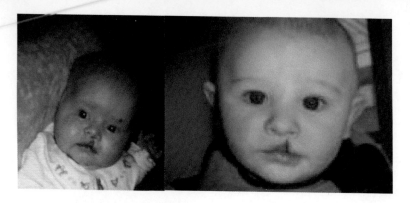

Isolated cleft palate can be missed

Small jaw – can cause tongue to fall backwards.

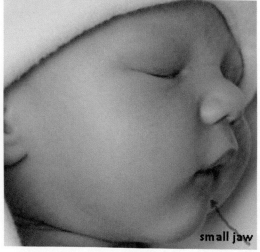

small jaw

Pierre Robin Anomaly

Pierre Robin anomaly, syndrome or sequence is a condition present at birth, in which the infant has a smaller-than-normal lower jaw, a tongue that falls back in the throat, and difficulty breathing. This means that it can result in the tongue choking the child in their sleep, there are many feeding difficulties for the child, and also the child may get inadequate oxygen throughout their daily routines.

The thing about Robin sequence is that since it is a genetic predisposition, there are many other symptoms that can follow along with it, including congestive heart failure, pulmonary hypertension, cleft palate, ear infections, and etc..

Without any prevention techniques, the children suffering from Robin sequence often need to go through oral (ENT) surgery in order to open up their airways more.

Referral is desired at 6-8 weeks check in view of possible problems although majority are identified at birth.

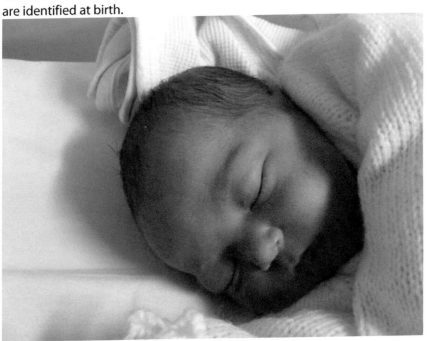

<u>Tongue Tie</u>

The frenulum of toungue
This usually doesn't cause problem but is a concern for parents. In past it was said to be associated with mild speech problems and dental hygiene

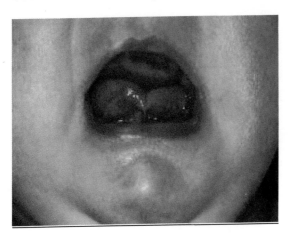

Neonatal jaundice and other disorders

Neonatal jaundice

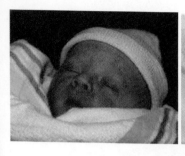 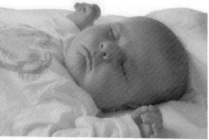

Jaundice is the yellow discolouration of the sclerae (whites of the eyes) and skin. It occurs in ¯60% of term babies and 80% of premature babies during the first week of life.

Jaundice is due to the deposition, in the tissues, of a yellow pigment called bilirubin. When the bilirubin exceeds a certain level, jaundice becomes obvious to the observer. Bilirubin is the end product of breakdown of red blood cells. This unconjugated form of bilirubin is then processed by the liver to become the conjugated form. Conjugated bilirubin is further processed in the gut and finally excreted from the body via the stool.

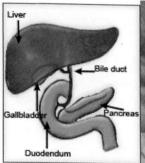 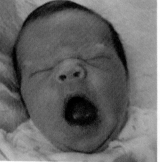

In healthy newborns, elevation of unconjugated bilirubin occurs commonly and is known as physiological jaundice. This occurs because:
- ➢ There is increased red blood cell (RBC) volume in newborns
- ➢ The life span of red blood cells (RBCs) is shorter in newborns as compared to adults
- ➢ The liver function is still immature

Physiological jaundice may occur from the 2nd day onwards and peaks by day 3 or 4 of life. Physiological jaundice, however, does not occur on the 1st day nor does it exceed beyond the 2nd week of life in term babies (or 3rd week in premature babies). If the jaundice persists beyond this period or if the level of jaundice is severe, then baby should be investigated for other underlying causes. **You will therefore not see a baby at 6-8 week baby check with physiological jaundice and a jaundice at this age needs further investigations.**

Causes of prolonged jaundice are:

> - Breast milk jaundice
> - Jaundice caused by liver disease- biliary atresia (blockage of bile flow)
> - Jaundice from other causes e.g. Haemolysis (red cell breakdown)- Blood group incompatibility between mother and baby — Rhesus; ABO ; Abnormal red blood cell (RBC) shape etc spherocytosis (rounded RBC); elliptocytosis (oval shaped RBC)
> - Jaundice caused by infection
> - Jaundice caused by hypothyroidism

Extravasated blood (bruises or blood clot) — e.g. cephalhaematoma (collection of blood below the membrane/layer which covers the skull bone) or subaponeurotic haemorrhage (collection of blood below the layer of muscle insertion). The blood within the swelling gets reabsorbed and broken into bilirubin, which subsequently causes jaundice. Both of these conditions are more likely to occur in babies delivered via forceps/vacuum extraction.

If all of the above medical conditions have been excluded and if it is unlikely that baby has any other less common conditions, there is a likelihood that baby has breast milk jaundice.

In breast milk jaundice, the jaundice usually appears at the end of/after the first week of life and may persist up to several weeks or even months. Breast milk jaundice occurs as a result of 'abnormal' milk content, which inhibits the bilirubin conjugation activity. Interruption of breastfeeding for 1-2 days with substitution of formula for breast milk (in moderately severe jaundice) will usually result in a rapid decline in bilirubin level after which breastfeeding may be resumed. Provided there are no additional risk factors, babies who have either physiological or breast milk jaundice will remain well and recover completely.

General assessment of baby with jaundice
> - Feeding history including whether breast or bottle-fed
> - Weight
> - liver enlargement
> - stool and urine colour
> - Inform parents of reason for blood tests

• Urine and stool colour-Community healthcare professionals should be aware of the importance of urine and stool colour:

> Normally a baby's urine is colourless
> Persistently yellow urine which stains the nappy can be a sign of liver disease
> Normally a baby's stools are green or yellow
> Persistently pale coloured stools may indicate liver disease

A jaundiced baby with pale stools and yellow urine can appear completely Healthy but this baby may have a potentially lethal liver disease.
If the stools and urine in a jaundiced baby are abnormal in colour, the baby should be referred to a paediatrician immediately.

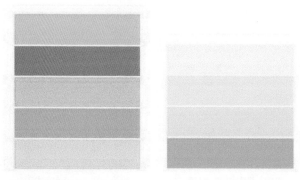

Healthy stool colours   **Suspicious stool colours**

Breast-fed babies may also have liver disease; be extra careful to check stools and urine.

Investigations in jaundice
> ABO group and rhesus status
> Coomb's test
> Blood film and reticulocyte count
> Total and direct bilirubin
> LFT
> Others as indicated

Treatment- Depends on the cause of jaundice and paediatricians will decide the management.

Hypoglycaemia mean low blood sugar and is the commonest neonatal metabolic disorder . It often has a non-specific presentation . Clinical features include lethargy, irritability, respiratory distress, tachycardia. Tachypnoea etc.

Predisposing factors are Diabetic mother , Prematurity / small for gestational age , Birth asphyxia , Sepsis, Hypothermia etc management is giving feed or sugar solution.

Module 5 Dysmorphic Features and congenital anomalies

Dysmorphic features

Dysmorphic features are abnormal facial and body features that can be subtle or obvious right from birth. The reasons can be genetic or constitutional. These can be classical of a syndrome or isolated abnormalities. These babies may need a detailed analysis of history and examination to identify a possible clue and extent of abnormality.

History Checklist for babies
➢ pregnancy history, noting particularly exposure to teratogens, amniotic fluid volume
➢ results of ultrasound and amniocentesis/CVS
➢ fetal movements
➢ maternal illness
➢ delivery history
➢ family history of abnormalities
➢ consanguinity

Examination Checklist
•**Growth- small for age**

•**Ectodermal features**
•skin – texture, colour, birthmarks, redundancy, defects
•hair - scalp hair and body hair: colour and distribution. anterior and posterior scalp hairline

•**Skull** -shape, symmetry,sutures (over-riding/normal/widely open) ,fontanelle size and number

•**Face-** Overall face shape, symmetry, facial muscle movement

•**Forehead region -** shape - (broad/bitemporal narrowing/tall)

•**Eyes-**
palpebral fissure length (short/long)
palpebral fissure slant (up/down) – upslant laterally in Downs syndrome, downslant laterally in Treacher Collin Syndrome
epicanthic folds - a fold of skin which arcs from below the eye into the upper lid

•**Midface region**

-nose-root ,bridge (depressed/prominent/broad) ,tip

- ears - position, shape and structure

Oral region
- mouth size and shape
- lip shape, thickness
- gum thickness
- philtrum definition and length
- jaw position (prognathia/ micrognathia)
- palate shape
- oral cavity - natal teeth/frenulum/tongue size and morphology

Hands and Feet
- overall shape and size of hand and foot
- digit number
- digit shape (e.g. clinodactyly) and length
- webbing between digits
- palmar, plantar and digit creases
- nail morphology

Joints and Skeleton
- contractures
- limb shortening
- joint range of movement
- soft tissue webbing across joints (pterygium)
- sternum length and shape (pectus carinatum/excavatum)
- shape of thoracic cage
- spine length, straight/curved
- neck length, webbing

Genitalia and Anus
- phallus size, morphology
- development of scrotum and palpation of testes
- development of labia
- position of anus relative to genitalia, patency of anus
- Investigations - when to do what?

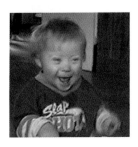
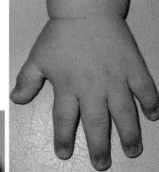
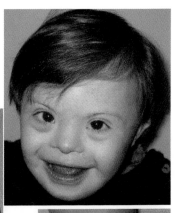
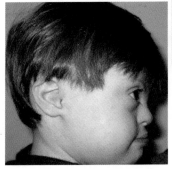
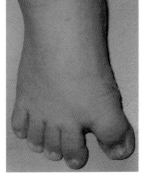
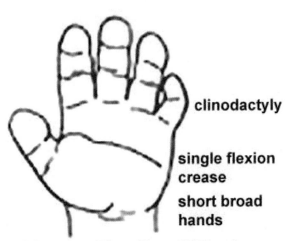

clinodactyly

single flexion
crease

short broad
hands

Trisomy 21 - Hand Features

Down's syndrome

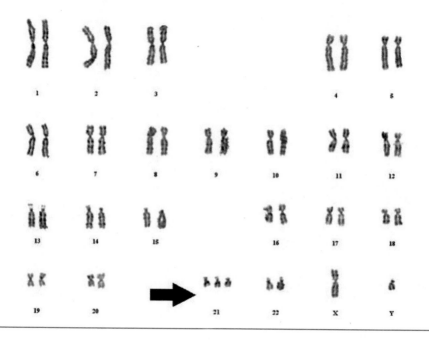

•Tests in the syndrome work-up
Renal USS
ECHO
Cranial USS
Eye examination
Skeletal Xrays
Chromosomes
FISH
Single gene
Biochemical tests

Communication Strategies with Parents

➢ Awkward
➢ Important to communicate
➢ Does the child resembles anyone in the family
➢ "Distinctive facial features"
➢ Dysmorphic features

Down's syndrome-Single palmer crease

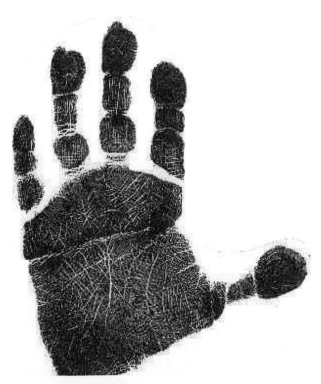

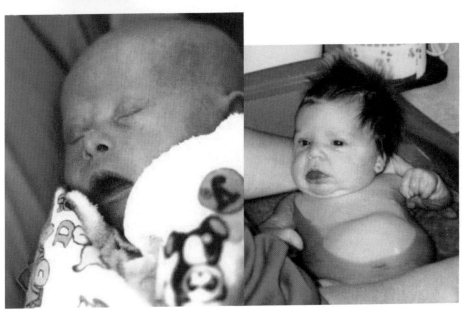

Congenital abnormalities

•Approximately 2% of live births have major congenital abnormality . Incidence is increased in pre-term and small for gestational age infants

•Malformation = disturbance of growth during embryogenesis

•Deformation = late change in previously normal structure due to intrauterine factors

Anatomical systems involved Teratogenesis or malformation

•Teratogen = drug, chemical or virus that can cause foetal malformation

•Act during critical period of foetal development

•Critical period varies between organs

—Brain   15-25 days

—Eye   25-40 days

—Heart   20-40 days

—Limb   24-36 days

Microbial agents as teratogens

•TORCHES - Rubella , Toxoplasmosis , Syphilis , Cytomegalovirus , Coxsackie B virus

Drugs as teratogens

➢ Hormones – progestogens, diethyl stilbeostrol, male sex hormones
➢ Antipsychotics – lithium, haloperidol, thalidomide
➢ Anticonvulsants – sodium valproate, carbamazepine, phenobarbitone
➢ Antimicrobials – tetracycline, chloramphenicol, amphotericin B
➢ Antineoplastics – alkylating agents, folic acid antagonists
➢ Anticoagulants – warfarin
➢ Antithyroid agents – carbimazole, propylthiouracil
➢ Others – toluene, alcohol, marijuana, narcotics

Sternomastoid tumours

It is lump on side of neck on middle third of sternomastoid muscle. It is a misnomer, not a tumour but results from muscle damage during labour. It presents with neck lump and torticollois away from affected side. Tilted head to one side i.e. torticollis may be resulting from muscular spasm (diferential diagnosis is baby tilting head trying to avoid double vision).

•Treatment should involve physiotherapy to correct the torticollois. Surgery to the lump is rarely required.

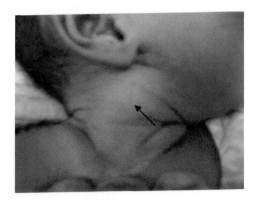

Cystic hygroma
It is another neck swelling . It often present in early childhood as expanding mass and contain clear fluid and transilluminate brightly. Large lesions can be diagnoses prenatally and can result in obstructed labour. It is due to lymphatic malformations resulting in multi-cystic mass and can be found else where, although 60% are found in neck region. Surgical excision is required although difficult and can result in a poor cosmetic result. Injection of sclerosing agents may be useful to try.

Branchial remnants
These neck swelling are rare and are foungd on anterior border of sternomastoid. Often bilateral and extend deep into neck, these are branchial sinuses and cysts arising from foetal second branchial sinus. Internal opening may occasionally found in tonsillar fossa .Treatment is by surgical excision

Neck lumps in children may be enlarged inflamed lymph nodes. Secondary to eczema or infection in and around neck or scalp.

Thyroglossal cysts are midline swellings in track of thyroid gland and move on protruding tongue.

•Dermoid cyst

Polydactily- can be soft tissue only or may contain bone or bony remnant.

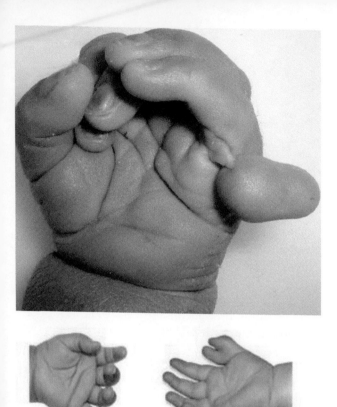

Presence of additional toes or fingers (Greek, poly = many, dactyly = digit) also called polydactylia or polydactylism. The condition is often treated surgically in the infant. Polydactyly can also be associated with a number of different syndromes including Greig cephalopolysyndactyly syndrome (GCPS).

There are also several forms of polydactyly including: preaxial polydactyly type-IV (PPD-IV) and postaxial polydactyly.

Preaxial polydactyly (PPD) has been shown as a defect in Sonic Hedgehog (Shh) expression. SHH is normally expressed specifically in the zone of polarizing activity (ZPA) located posteriorly in the limb bud and is expressed in an additional ectopic site (at the anterior margin) in a mouse model of this disorder.

Syndactily

Fusion of fingers or toes (Greek, syn = together, dactyly = digit) which may be single or multiple and may affect: skin only, skin and soft tissues or skin, soft tissues and bone. The condition is unimportant in toes but disabling in fingers and requires operative separation and is frequently inherited as an autosomal dominant. The presence of this additional "webbing" reflects preservation of the developmental tissues that in normal development are removed by programmed cell death (apotosis).

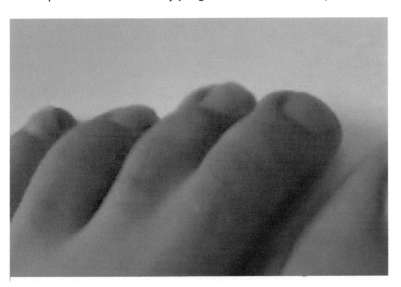

Talipes Equinovarus

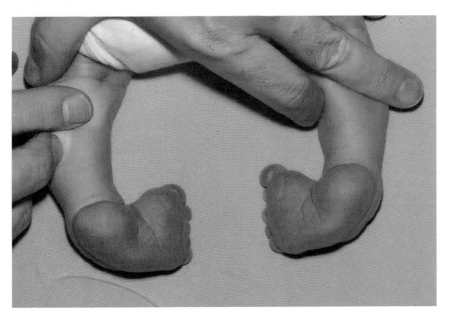

Abnormality of the lower limb which begins in the embryonic period (first trimester of pregnancy) resulting in the foot is then turned inward and downward at birth, described as "club foot".

Occurs in approximately 1 in 1,000 births, postnatally it affects how children walk on their toes with the foot pointed downward like a horse (Latin, talipes = ankle bone, pes = foot, equinus = horse).

Can also occur in asociation with other syndromes. For example, camptomelic dysplasia, an extremely rare (2 per million live births) lethal congenital bony dysplasia which can be detected by ultrasound (25 weeks) visible as anterior bowing of long bones.

Visual Examination in babies and blindness

General Eye Examination
- ➤ General inspection of eye
- ➤ Assessment of eye movement
- ➤ Pupil and reaction to light
- ➤ Red reflex
- ➤ Ophthalmoscope handling
- ➤ Assessment of vision

Hold your face nearly 30-50 cm from baby's face and grab the attention. See if the baby can focus on your face. When baby focus, move your face side to side and see if the baby moves eyes in the same direction.

General inspection of eyes- you will see eye lids, eye brows, eye lashes, cornea, white sclera, iris etc as noted in figure. Sub-conjunctival haemorrhages are blood spots in eye , are common findings and may be found in as many as 20-30% of newborn infants. It generally is present right from birth and reflect the significant pressure inherent in molding of the head as it passes the birth canal.

Colobomas (missing pieces of the iris) are most commonly located in the lower half and point in the direction of the nose. Too small or too large corneas may be isolated findings, or may be part of a general malformation (microphthalmus or macrophthalmus). Any significant malformation of the eyes should be referred to an opthamologist.

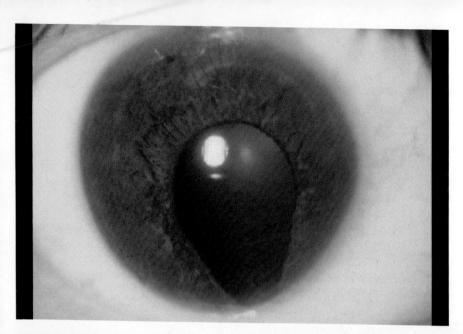

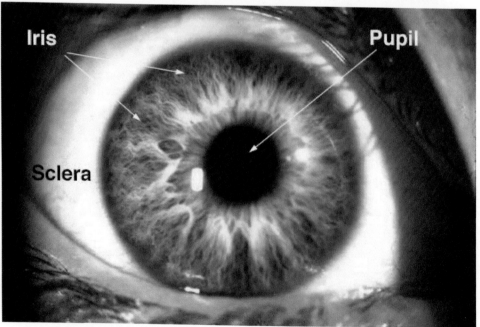

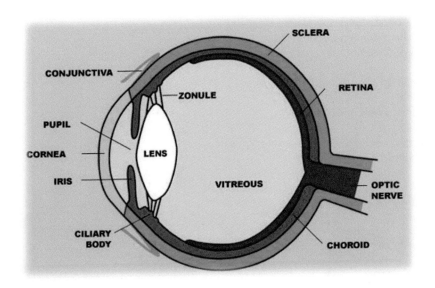

Ophthalmoscope handling Directions

It's important to have confidence in handling ophthalmoscope and get the correct information using this equipment. The steps to using the ophthalmoscope are:

1. Screw the head onto the power base if not connected already.
Match the notches in the Ophthalmoscope head with those on the power source (see illustration)

Press down until notches mesh
Twist clockwise
Pull gently to see if head is secure

2. Turn the ophthalmoscope on

Press red button on the top rim of the power source
handle in a downward
direction
Twist the button clockwise around the rim. You should be able to see the
light in the palm of your hand when you point the narrow end toward your palm.

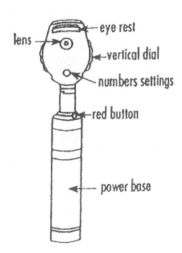

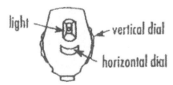

other side of ophthalmoscope head

3. View the eye with the ophthalmoscope
Turn the vertical dial with your thumb until it is on the "0" setting
(see illustration)
Find the "large circle of light" by turning the horizontal dial with your
thumb (see illustration)
View both eyes at same time to assess red reflex

*Important: Keep a distance of about 12 inches between you and the child. Dim the
room light for better view.
Red reflux

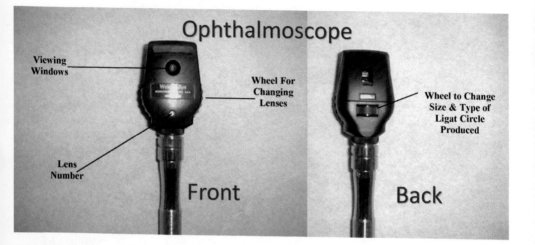

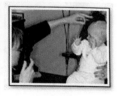 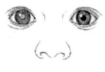

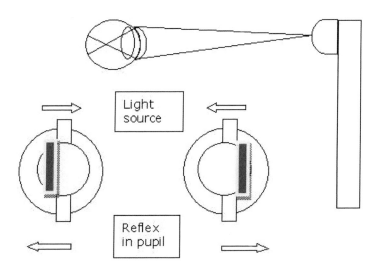

White pupil may indicate cataract, tumor, inflammation, or detached retina.

Complete or partial absence of pupil is to be noted as it may be associate with other anomalies.

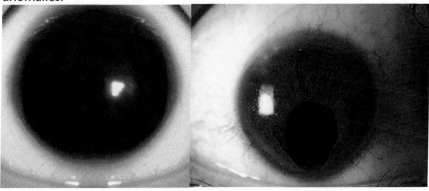

How to examine eyes at the 6-8 week check
Inspection
Assessment of vision

c) Assessment of Eye movements
Fixing and following of interesting objects
- ➢ Turn head to light
- ➢ Vestibular ocular reflex-Rotate infant's head gently side to side and back forward, up and down to elicit eye movements
- ➢ Squint will have limitation due to muscle imbalance.

d) **Pupil**- see the colour, normally black. If white, suspect cataract or retinoblastoma. Pupillary responses to light- constriction – shine light in one eye – that pupil constricts (the other pupil may also constrict and it is called indirect or consensual response) .

e) *The red reflex*

It is an important test to make sure baby has clear media for light passage right through to back of eye i.e. retina. Principle is that the ophthalmoscope shines light into eye and it goes through cornea, lens and vitreous liquid to retina and gets reflected to be seen in as bright orange , red or yellow area in pupil. It is in some way similar to "red eye" as seen in many flash photos. The procedure consist of holding ophthalmoscope close to your eye and shine a light into baby's eye from nearly half a meter away. You will see a red reflection whilst looking down ophthalmoscope(may be orange or yellow). Absence indicate blockage in media i.e. corneal opacity, cataract, retinoblastoma etc and is always pathological.

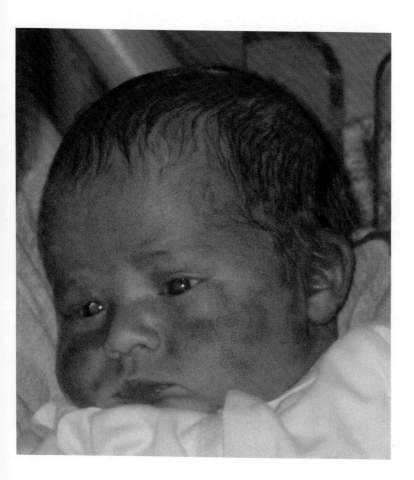

The Leukocoric pupil:

Although every newborn receives a baseline exam after birth by paediatrician or qualified midwife checking for a good red-reflex off the retina, it is important to check it again. Leukocoria describes a white-colored pupil. This finding should concern you and requires an ophthalmology consult as the causes may be serious. Potential causes of leukocoria are:

1. Congenital Cataract
2. Retinoblastoma
3. ROP (retinopathy of prematurity)

There are many other causes for a white pupil, such as persistent hyperplastic primary vitreous, but let's focus on above three, the third one would have been dealt in neonatal unit and mother would be aware.

Congenital Cataract

A cataract in a newborn can occur by several mechanisms. They can be idiopathic, genetic, from metabolic disorders, child abuse trauma, or caused by one of the maternal TORCH infections during fetal development. Whatever the cause, it is important to remove these cataracts as soon as possible as they are amblyogenic and will lead to permanent vision loss from visual neglect. Replacing a lens is tricky, however, as babies are tiny, generate an impressive inflammatory response, and their "prescription" is still changing as the eye continues to grow. The cataract is removed as soon as possible, but often the lens implant can be placed at a later date - parents have to deal with aphakic contact lens or thick glasses in the meantime.

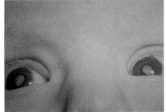

congenital cataract both eyes - rubella

Retinoblastoma

Retinoblastoma is a tumor of the primitive retinal photoreceptors. The tumor grows on the retina and forms a white or cream-colored mass that can completely fill the eye, creating a white iris, and often a retinal detachment.

Retinoblastoma is the most common primary malignant ocular tumor in children. That being said, the cancer is still very rare, with only 250-500 new cases reported in the

United States each year. You don't want to miss this one, though, as failure to diagnose RB results in the death of a child.

These children are under 4 years of age, with the average age of diagnosis 18 months. There are different types of RB, and the tumor can arise from a random somatic mutation or develop along several germline inheritance patterns.

Treatment modalities are many, but decisive treatment often involves enucleation (removal) of the entire eye to avoid seeding tumor cells into the orbit. The tumor spreads by extension down the optic nerve toward the brain so it is important to get a good optic nerve section upon removal with careful microscopic evaluation for margin involvement. The overall survival rate in the US is very good, approaching 90%, but only if the tumor is recognized early.

Retinopathy of Prematurity
ROP is an important disease process that is commonly found in neonatal ICUs. Here's how ROP works:
The retinal blood supply begins formation around week 16 of gestation, with retinal vessels springing forth from the optic disk and spreading outwards in an expanding fan toward the edges of the retina. By the 8th (36 weeks) month this vasculature has reached the nasal retinal-edge, and within a few more months the whole retinal blood supply has formed 360 degrees.

Everything sounds good, right? Well, problems can occur if a child is born premature. With premature eye metabolism, areas of peripheral retina that haven't yet developed blood supply can become ischemic. Ischemic retina produces VEGF with resulting neovascularization. These neovascular vessels can bleed, create traction, and eventually retinal detachment. A leukocoric "white pupil" can result if the retinal detachment is big enough. The more premature a child is born, the more likely this unfortunate sequence of events is to occur. For this reason, children born under 32 weeks or less than 1,500 grams are screened to insure their retina is forming properly.

We treat these kids in a similar fashion as proliferative diabetic retinopathy in adults – PRP laser or cryotherapy is used to ablate the peripheral ischemic retina in an attempt to shut down excess VEGF production.

Fundoscopy is difficult in newborn babies and is not required routinely. It is to see the close view of the retina and should be done by the people experienced in doing so based on need. If there is doubt about vision or eye abnormality you ring or refer to paediatrician, or ophthalmologist in conjunction with GP.

Practical – Examination of eyes – opening eyes may be a talk in 6-8 week babies. One trick is to lift the baby and rotate gently side to side. It may send a stimulus to brain and in many cases babies open eyes.

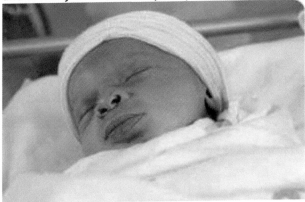

ABNORMALITIES in vision

The visual Pathway involve rays coming from object to front of eye, getting through cornea, transparent liquid that bathe eye , lens and back of eye(retina). The visual message about object is here converted into a nerve impulse to travel through nerves into skull and brain to reach the optic cortex (area of brain that interprets the object by converting nerve impulse back into visual message).Any problem in the pathway any where can result into visual impairment.

Maturation of vision-Newborns baby has poor vision as compared to adult, the acuity is 6/200. The acuity is 6/60 by 3 months and 6/6 by 3 years which is similar to adult.

Presentations of visual impairment

- Lack of eye contact
- Visual inattention
- Random eye movements
- No social smile by 6 weeks
- Nystagmus
- Squint
- Photophobia
- No red reflex

Visual handicap may mask the true intellectual ability of child and appear to make developmental delay worse

Causes of visual impairment – general mechanism

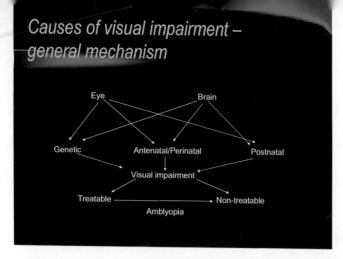

Childhood blindness – It is interesting to know that 50 million people are blind world-wide and 1.4 million children are blind worldwide. In UK in 2000 there were 439 newly diagnosed children with visual impairment and ¾ of these had other disabilities. 60% of these had prenatal cause (different to developing world). 24,000 under 16s in UK sight problems, 60% attend a mainstream school and 60% have SSEN.

Causes of visual impairment – general mechanism

Amblyopia (commonly resulting from "lazy eye") may cause Permanent loss of visual acuity in an eye that has not received a clear image. It affects 2-3% children and usually affects only one eye. It is caused by any interference with visual development. Once interference is removed vision may develop, however after 7 years age unlikely to be improvement, hence earlier underlying cause treated, the better the prognosis.

Important treatable causes of amblyopia in a 6-8 weeks baby can be obscured visual field e.g. Corneal opacity ,Lens opacity (Cataract),Retinoblastoma, Large haemangioma covering eye etc. The doctors may treat underlying cause and do patching to allow development of vision in eye that has gone lazy.

Cavernous haemangioma (Strawberry mark) may grow and cover eye

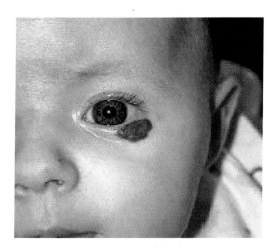

Retinoblastoma- *it i*s a tumour of retina, Hereditary or acquired, ca be picked up by absent red reflex, or squint. Treatment is surgery and goal is to preserve vision. If diagnosed early 95% survival rate

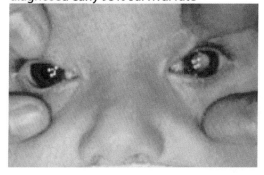

Retinopathy of prematurity

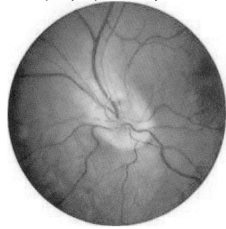

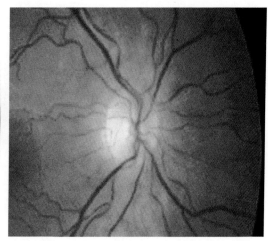

•*Central Causes for blindness in bay can be* Secondary to hypoxic injury – term baby with perinatal brain injury or following intraventricular haemorrhage in preterm. Brain or optic nerve / pathway problem or Congenital brain abnormality.

<u>*Sight threatening conjunctivitis -*</u> This may occur in neonatal period and is due to bacterial infection , the one due to gonococcal infection is rapidly progressive to cause blindness. Antibiotic treatment is required systemically so do get second opinion as soon as possible.

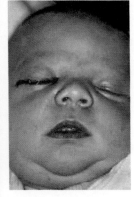

Drooping eye lid - May be an inflammation, which is an emergency if it happens suddenly and the lid is red and hot. Also may indicate muscle weakness and need referral due to risk to the vision.

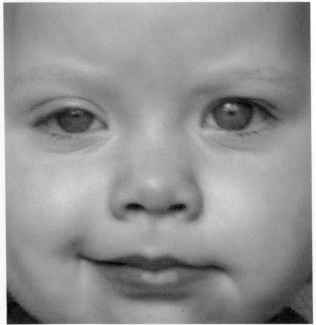

Blocked naso-lacrimal duct

There is a gland under the upper eye lid that produces secretions all the time and keep eye moist. This secretions is constantly drained by tear duct to the nose. There is an opening of the tear duct connection in both upper and lower lid and there is a kind of bag where these join main tear duct called naso-lacrimal sac. This may get infected leading to redness and swelling medial to eye. It will need treatment with antibiotic. It may however just become swollen when there is blockage of tear duct which is much more common and a gentle massage of the area may clear the blockage. It may cause excessive tear or watering of eye due to blockage. If it doesn't get clear with massage , it may need probing or operation.

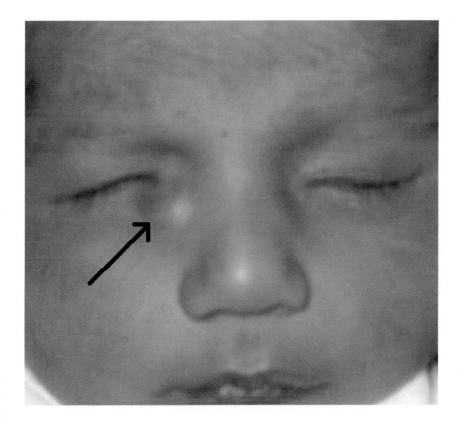

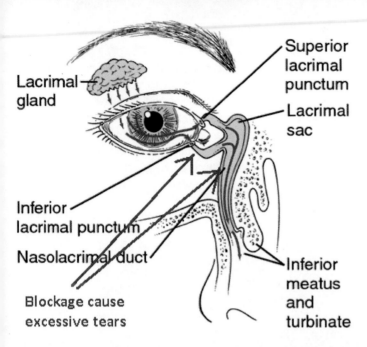

Lacrimal gland

Superior lacrimal punctum

Lacrimal sac

Inferior lacrimal punctum

Nasolacrimal duct

Blockage cause excessive tears

Inferior meatus and turbinate

Nystagmus A dancing eye movement or eye jiggle is a sign of disease of the nervous system anywhere between the eyes and the brain. Any baby who does not look at you despite of effort to engage need a senior opinion.

Unequal pupil- One pupil larger. May be a sign of nerve damage which is visible in one eye.

The causes of blindness can be outside eye, with in eye and in brain along the pathway shown below.

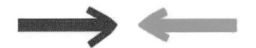

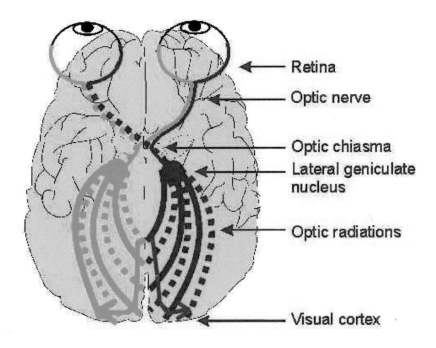

- Retina
- Optic nerve
- Optic chiasma
- Lateral geniculate nucleus
- Optic radiations
- Visual cortex

Squint

Can be normal in first few weeks of life due to immaturity of balance of muscles controlling eye movements, however if vision is normal parents can be reassured and it should be followed up. If there is problem in vision , advice of specialist should be sought.

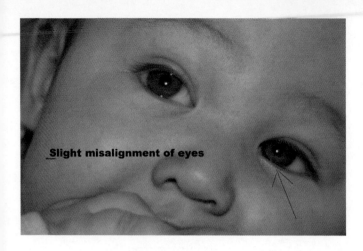

Slight misalignment of eyes

Shaken Baby Syndrome and child protection issues

Child safe gauarding is an extremely important issue and we all should try to pick up early indications from history and examination.

Sheken baby syndrome is a condition that can cause serious brain problem and is preventable.

New babies cry a lot - on average three hours a day, and often for no apparent reason. Some babies cry significantly more than this! Frustrated caregivers may pick up the child and shake it if suitably irate. This shaking can become a reinforcing response as the infant becomes somnolent afterwards and stops crying, exactly the response the caregiver was hoping for. Infants are predisposed to physical damage from shaking as they have big heads and weak neck muscles. As the head whiplashes back and forth, the acceleration and deceleration forces traumatize the brain in a big way. Biological fathers and boyfriends are the most common perpetrators of this behavior, but anyone can be the attacker – this phenomenon spares no ethnicity, religion, culture, or social class.

These children can be of any age in first year although usually 5 to 10 months of age and present with sleepiness, seizures or coma. The classic triad of exam findings include:

1. Intracranial hemorrhage: usually a subdural hemorrhage secondary to tearing of the small bridging veins between the dura mater and arachnoid.
2. Brain swelling: from shearing forces, diffuse axonal damage, secondary edema, and infarction.
3. Retinal hemorrhages: specific findings (see below).

The child can also have other physical findings such as bruising of the body trunk (where the shaker grips the child) and fractures of the skull, long bones, or ribs. Remember: be suspicious for abuse when you see many bone fractures at different stages of healing.

CT scan of shaken baby with intracranial bleed show sub-dural haemorrgahe as below.

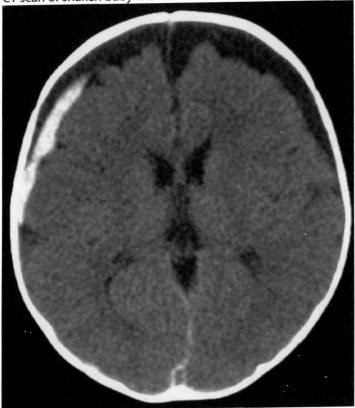

Retinal Findings:

An ophthalmologist needs to be called in for any case of potential shaken baby to evaluate the retina. These kids have specific retinal hemorrhages that aren't really seen in any other condition:

1. Large retinal hemorrhages located in all quadrants of the eye, located in all layers of the retina (subretinal, intraretinal, and preretinal).
2. Retinoschisis cavities. A schisis is a split between layers of the retina, and is very suspicious for abuse in this age group.

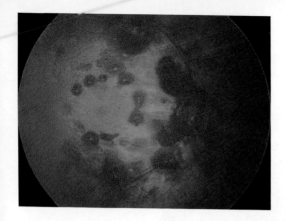

It's imperative to write a descriptive note in the chart (have the attending write this note for litigation reasons) and document any bleeding with fundus photography. You want to take these photos soon, as hemorrhages can resolve in only a few days!

What about other causes of retinal bleeding?

Studies have found that household injuries, such as a fall from caregiver's arms or furniture doesn't usually cause significant retinal hemorrhage. Birth trauma can cause mild retinal bleeding but this is usually limited and resolves in the first few months. CPR with chest compressions rarely causes significant hemorrhaging. The hemorrhages in SBS are impressive and similar retinal bleeding isn't seen except with big trauma such as a high-speed car wreck or a multi-story fall.

Be sure to look for any coagulopathy with basic lab testing, including CBC, coags, platelet count and bleeding time.

Prognosis:
While a third of these babies have no long term sequela, the long-term prognosis is generally bad. Twenty percent of these abused children die outright and the remaining kids end up with life-changing developmental problems, mental retardation, blindness, paralysis, and behavioral changes.

Hearing problems

Hearing problems in 6-8 week check are not so common, however has significant implications. Early detection and referral is desirable although a majority of abnormalities are now picked at neonatal screening programme.

Objectives
- Examination of ears
- General idea of hearing mechanism
- Assessment of hearing
- Common causes of hearing impairmant

Ear is one of very important sensory organ and problems can be devastating. It is interesting that majority of hearing abnormalities are picked up be the neonatal hearing screening and the suspicious cases are recalled. It is however still important to have some sense of hearing at in 6-8 week baby check. There may be congenital abnormalities of the ear or the hearing mechanism.

How do we hear

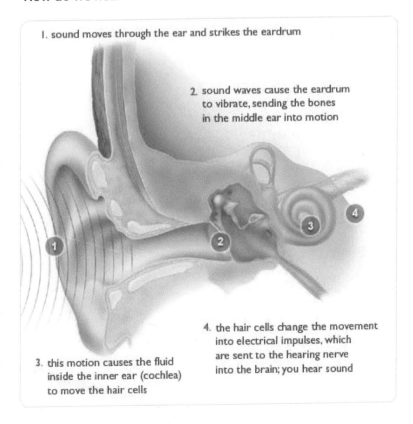

1. sound moves through the ear and strikes the eardrum

2. sound waves cause the eardrum to vibrate, sending the bones in the middle ear into motion

3. this motion causes the fluid inside the inner ear (cochlea) to move the hair cells

4. the hair cells change the movement into electrical impulses, which are sent to the hearing nerve into the brain; you hear sound

- Anatomy
- Physiology of hearing
- Hearing loss
- Checklist of hearing
- Hearing tests
- Referrals

- Sound consists of vibrations of air in the form of waves.
- The ear is able to pick up these vibrations and convert them into electrical signals that are sent to the brain.

- In the brain, these signals are translated into meaningful information, such as language or music with qualities like volume and pitch. The volume of sound is measured in decibels (dB).

- Loudness is measured in decibels (dB)
- This is the force of sound waves against the ear
- The louder the sound the more decibels
- Humans cannot hear sounds of every frequency. The range of hearing for a healthy young person is 20 to 20,000 hertz

Frequency (Hz)
- Number of vibrations per second = frequency
- varies for each sound and is measured in hertz.
- One hertz = one vibration per second.
- A sound with a low frequency will have a low pitch, such as a human's heartbeat.
- A sound with a high frequency will have a high pitch, such as a dog whistle.

Checklist for reaction to sound
Shortly after birth – a baby

- Is startled by a sudden loud noise such as a hand clap or a door slamming
- Blinks or opens eyes widely to such sounds or stops sucking or starts to cry

Checklist for reaction to sound
1 month – a baby

- Starts to notice sudden prolonged sounds like the noise of a vacuum cleaner and may turn towards the noise
- Pauses and listens to the noises when they begin

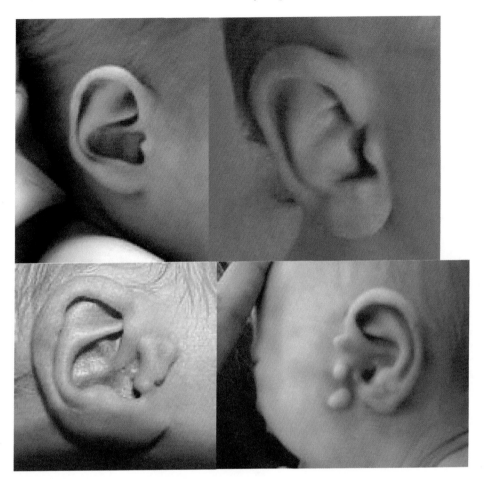

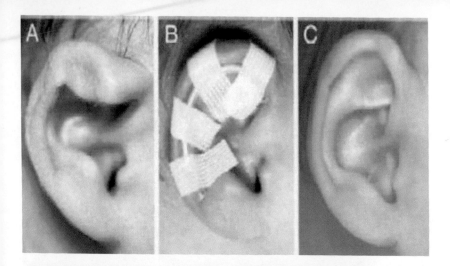

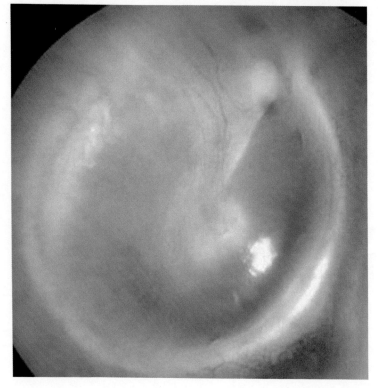

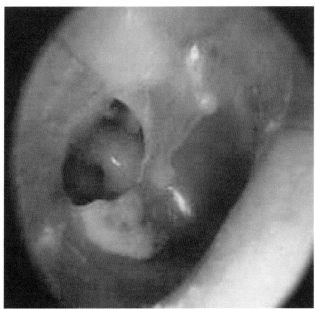

Hearing Screening
•Done at birth or within the first few weeks of life
•Otoacoustic Emissions
•AABR

Hearing loss
•There are many possible causes of hearing loss. These can be divided into two basic types, called conductive and sensorineural hearing loss.
Conductive hearing loss
•is caused by anything that interferes with the transmission of sound from the outer to the inner ear.

• Possible causes include:
➢   middle ear infections (otitis media)
➢   collection of fluid in the middle ear ("glue ear" in children)
➢   blockage of the outer ear (by wax)
➢   damage to the eardrum by infection or an injury

Sensorineural hearing loss
•is due to damage to the pathway for sound impulses from the hair cells of the inner ear to the auditory nerve and the brain.

•otosclerosis, a condition in which the ossicles of the middle ear become immobile because of growth of the surrounding bone

•rarely, rheumatoid arthritis affects the joints between the ossicles.

Possible causes include

➢ viral infections of the inner ear (mumps or measles)
➢ viral infections of the auditory nerve (such as mumps and rubella)
➢ certain drugs e.g. some antibiotics, which can affect the hair cells
➢ infections or inflammation of the brain or brain covering - e.g. meningitis
➢ Inherited causes

Referral

➢ If parents do not attend the outpatient appointment
➢ Any babies born at home
➢ Babies moving into the area
➢ Concerns about the child's hearing

Nervous system

"Normal full-term newborns lie in a symmetrical position with limbs semiflexed and legs partially abducted at the hip. The head is slightly flexed and positioned in the midline or turned to one side. Normal newborns have spontaneous motor activity of flexion and extension, alternating between the arms and legs. The forearms supinate with flexion at the elbow and pronate with extension. The fingers are usually flexed in a tight fist, but may extend in slow athetoid posturing movements. Low-amplitude and high-frequency tremors of the arms and legs called jitteriness may be seen with vigorous crying and even at rest during the first few days of life."

In the newborn, flexor tone is predominate. After the first few weeks, the flexor tone is less. Passive range of motion is still met with resistance but with the appropriate amount. The hand pulled across the body to the opposite shoulder still does not extend beyond the shoulder.

Although this baby's resting posture shows some flexion of the lower extremities, the upper and lower extremities are in more extension than flexion. The hips are fully abducted and there is little spontaneous movement. There are some gravity opposing movements but they are infrequent. If the baby has a "flat on the mat" appearance it reflects low tone and possible weakness.

Testing muscle tone and posture is a part of baby check, for detection of any abnormality (video can be viewed at 6-8 weeks baby check eTrainingskill.com)

Floppy infant

Hypotonia, also called floppy infant syndrome or infantile hypotonia, is a condition of decreased muscle tone. The low muscle tone can be caused by a variety of conditions and is often indicative of the presence of an underlying central nervous system disorder, genetic disorder, or muscle disorder. Muscle tone is the amount of tension or resistance to movement in a muscle.

It is not the same as muscle weakness, which is a reduction in the strength of a muscle, but it can co-exist with muscle weakness. Muscle tone indicates the ability of a muscle to respond to a stretch. For example, if the flexed arm of a child with normal tone is quickly straightened, the flexor muscle of the arm (biceps) will quickly contract in response. Once the stimulus is removed, the muscle then relaxes and returns to its normal resting state. A child with low muscle tone has muscles that are slow to start a muscle contraction. Muscles contract very slowly in response to a stimulus and cannot maintain a contraction for as long as a normal muscle. Because low-toned muscles do not fully contract before they again relax, they remain loose and very stretchy, never achieving their full potential of sustaining a muscle contraction over time.

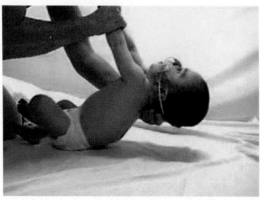
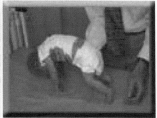

Hypotonic infants, therefore, have a typical **"floppy"** appearance. They rest with their elbows and knees loosely extended, while infants with normal muscle tone tend to have flexed elbows and knees. Head control is usually poor or absent in the floppy infant with the head falling to the side, backward, or forward. Infants with normal tone can be lifted by placing hands under their armpits, but hypotonic infants tend to slip between the hands as their arms rise unresistingly upward. While most children tend to flex their elbows and knees when resting, hypotonic children hang their arms and legs limply by their sides. Infants with this condition often lag behind in reaching the fine and gross motor developmental milestones that enable infants to hold their heads up when placed on the stomach, balance themselves, or get into a sitting position and remain seated without falling over. Hypotonia is also characterized by problems with mobility and posture, lethargy, weak ligaments and joints, and poor reflexes. Since the muscles that support the bone joints are so soft, there is a tendency for hip, jaw, and neck dislocations to occur. Some hypotonic children also have trouble feeding and are unable to suck or chew for long periods. Others may also have problems with speech or exhibit shallow breathing. Hypotonia does not, however, affect intellect.

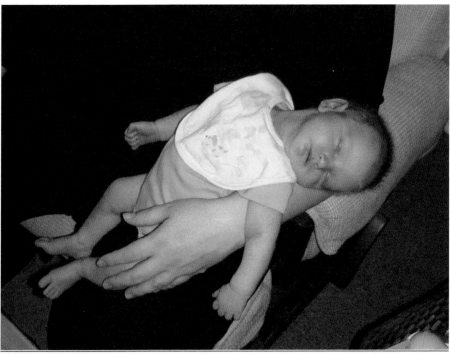

Causes

- o Down syndrome: a chromosome abnormality, usually due to an extra copy of the twenty-first chromosome.
- o Spinal muscular atrophy type 1 (Werdnig-Hoffman): a group of inherited diseases causing progressive muscle degeneration and weakness, eventually leading to death.
- o Congenital hypothyroidism: a disorder that results from decreased thyroid hormone production.
- o Prader-Willi syndrome: a congenital disease characterized by obesity, severe hypotonia, and decreased mental capacity
- o Kernicterus: also called Rh incompatibility, a condition that develops when there is a difference in Rh blood type between that of the mother (Rh negative) and that of the fetus (Rh positive).
- o Cerebellar ataxia: a movement disorder which with its sudden onset, often following an infectious viral disease, causes hypotonia.

Typical medical history questions include:

- ➤ When was the hypotonia first noticed?
- ➤ Was it present at birth?
- ➤ Did it start suddenly or gradually?
- ➤ Is the hypotonia always the same or does it seem worse at certain times?
- ➤ Is the child limp all over or only in certain areas?

> What other symptoms are present?

No specific treatment is required to treat mild congenital hypotonia, but children with this problem may periodically need treatment for common conditions associated with hypotonia, such as recurrent joint dislocations. Treatment programs to help increase muscle strength and sensory stimulation programs are developed once the cause of the child's hypotonia is established. Physiotherapy may be required. All such patients need to be referred to paediatrician for further assessment.

Asymmetrical movements of the arms and legs at any time should alert clinician to the possibility of central or peripheral neurologic defects, birth injuries, or congenital anomalies.

Meningitis

Meningitis is inflammation of the linings surrounding the brain and can be caused by bacteria, viruses or fungus (bacterial and viral being more common) Viral Meningitis is the most prevalent, however is rarely life threatening.

Bacterial Meningitis on the other hand can prove to be fatal and requires urgent treatment with antibiotics. It is predominantly caused by meningococcal bacteria but can be caused by pneumococcal, Hib
It can present with a 'flu-like symptoms, poor feeding, Vomiting , Drowsiness
Typical features are non-blanching rash   , bulging fontanelle

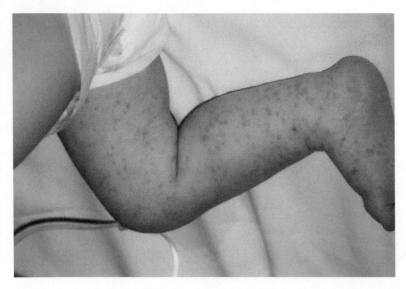

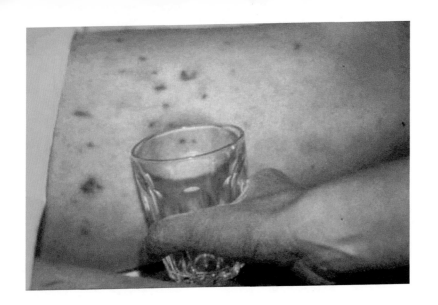

Developmental assessment

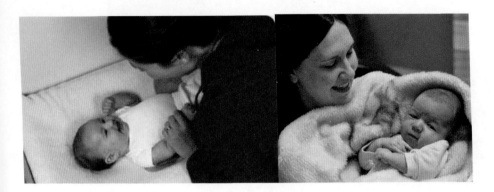

Developmental Milestones by the End of the First Month

Movement
- ➤ Makes jerky, quivering arm thrusts
- ➤ Brings hands within range of eyes and mouth
- ➤ Moves head from side to side while lying on stomach
- ➤ Head flops backward if unsupported
- ➤ Keeps hands in tight fists
- ➤ Strong reflex movements

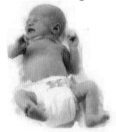

Visual
- ➤ Focuses 8 to 12 inches away
- ➤ Eyes wander and occasionally cross
- ➤ Prefers black-and-white or high-contrast patterns
- ➤ Prefers the human face to all other patterns

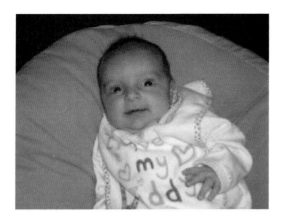

Hearing
> ➢ Hearing is fully mature
> ➢ Recognizes some sounds
> ➢ May turn toward familiar sounds and voices

Smell and Touch
> ➢ Prefers sweet smells
> ➢ Avoids bitter or acidic smells
> ➢ Recognizes the scent of his own mother's breast milk
> ➢ Prefers soft to coarse sensations
> ➢ Dislikes rough or abrupt handling
> ➢ Developmental Health Watch

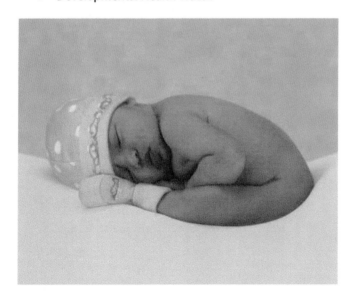

If, during the 6-8 weeks baby check you notice any of the following signs, discuss with GP and consider referral to a pediatrician.

- ➢ Sucks poorly and feeds slowly
- ➢ Doesn't blink when shown a bright light
- ➢ Doesn't focus and follow a nearby object moving side to side
- ➢ Rarely moves arms and legs; seems stiff
- ➢ Seems excessively loose in the limbs, or floppy
- ➢ Lower jaw trembles constantly, even when not crying or excited
- ➢ Doesn't respond to loud sounds

FAILURE to Thrive

Failure to thrive (FTT) is a medical term which denotes poor weight gain and physical growth failure. The term has been in medical use for over a century, however **faltering growth** is now the more politically correct term. Babies lose weight in first few days but regain birth weight by 10 days age. Failure to thrive is progressive weight drop across centile lines on growth chart.

Check for the milk intake, presence of diarrhea, vomitings, perianal rash, eczema, and any abnormality on systemic examination.

If you are a heath visitor, keep a close eye on baby and monitor weight weekly, however if there is a sharp drop, arrange referral to paediatrician.

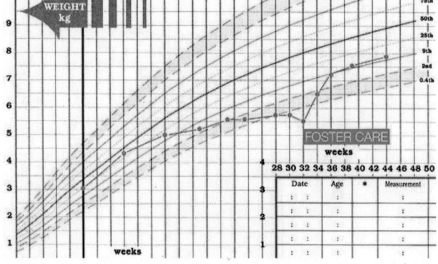

Cardiovascular problems

Heart sounds and murmurs

Heart works amazingly constantly and tirelessly 24/7, beating nearly 70-100 times a minute. There is a system for its working controlling flow of blood through valves and vessels and as a result there are heart sounds produced. These can be heard with stethoscope and a careful attention will help health visitors or nurse practitioners to differentiate different sounds.

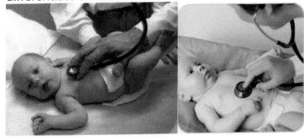

When we start to touch a baby, it is our preference to perform the cardiac examination first. This is because reliable auscultation of the heart is the one part of your total examination of the infant which is most dependent on having a quiet baby. However, if the baby is screaming, you can either delay the cardiac exam until later in the process, or you can swaddle the baby with a blanket and cradle/rock it in your arms, as this will often soothe her/him.

Observe the chest for any signs of palpitations or visible pulses. Remember to warm the stethoscope e.g. by holding it between your hands - a cold instrument is more likely to startle the baby.

Start by localizing the heart sounds. Are they more prominent on right or left (normally hear t is on left side so the sounds are more prominent on left) Check what is the heart rate? Auscultation of an infant's heart is quite difficult, and requires a lot of practice, particularly because heart rate is faster than adults.

The most obvious of the heart sounds are the first and second sounds, called S1 and S2. The period between first and second sound is called systole and that between second and first sound is called diastole.

These sounds are heard with a stethoscope. The stethoscope has a diaphragm and may have a bell . The diaphragm is used most of time. (Bell is better for listening to low frequency sounds, while the diaphragm transmits higher frequency sounds.)

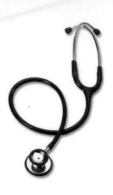
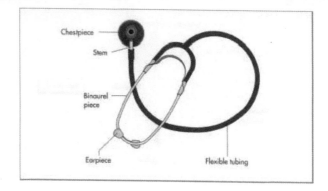

Angle the earpieces forward to match the direction of your external ear canal.

Place the diaphragm on the chest around nipple area to listen.
Ensure that you can hear the heart sounds **"lub-dup"** each time

First Heart Sound: S1 "lub" . This is caused by the closure of the mitral and tricuspid valves just before ventricular systole (when contraction of the ventricles expels blood out of the heart)

Second Heart Sound: S2 "dup". This is caused by closure of the aortic and pulmonary valves at the end of systole as the ventricles begin to relax (diastole).

The diagram below demonstrates this timing using standard shorthand notation derived from phonocardiography.

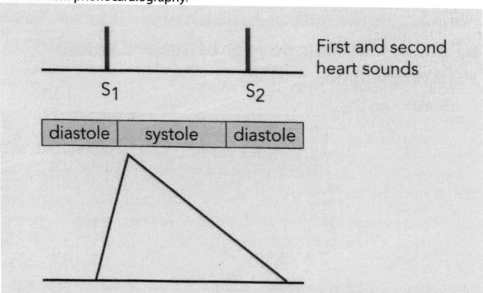

These heart sounds S1 and S2 are created by the near-instantaneous closing of two separate valves in heart. Generally, each of these is heard as single sound but some times they are split due to change in blood flow pattern. Some times a third and fourth heart sound is also heard, which again indicates change in pattern of blood flow and opening or closing of heart valves.

When listening to a patient's heart, the cadence of the beat will usually distinguish S1 from S2. Because diastole takes about twice as long as systole, there is a longer pause between S2 and S1 than there is between S1 and S2. However, rapid heart rates can shorten diastole to the point where it is difficult to discern which is S1 and which is S2. For this reason, it is important to always palpate the chest or the pulse at elbow when auscultating. The heart sound you hear when you first feel the pulse is S1, and when the pulse disappears is S2.

Normal sounds have no murmurs - just S1 and S2 - "lub dup" pattern.
ASD has characteristic S2 fixed split (two parts in the sound).
Innocent murmurs amplitude (intensity) is relatively small.

With some training (achieved by repetitive listening of audio tracks in resources section) it will become easier to detect these abnormalities by locking ear to their characteristic high frequency "wooosh" or "wooop" sound that is also of high intensity.

Normal = [LUP_DUP]
Innocent = [LUP_SHH_DUP]
VSD = [SHHHHH_DU_DRR]
AS = [RRR_drup or RRR_DHH]
PS = [LU_RRR_DUPdup]
ASD=[LUP_DU_DUP or LUH_RRR_DU_DUP]]

ASD murmur has lower intensity, but characteristic fixed split S2 sound. It
has acoustic perception of "drupp" or "dudup" (LUH_RRR_DU_DUP).
These simple observations may help to rule in abnormality. Innocent murmurs
are comparatively soft and often have musical- "twangy" quality.

When a valve is stenotic or damaged, the abnormal turbulent flow of blood produces a murmur which can be heard during the normally quiet times of systole or diastole. This murmur may not be audible over all areas of the chest, and it is useful to note where it is heard best.

As a health visitor or nurse practitioner it is enough to find an abnormal heart sound or murmur and you must seek advice of a senior medical professional. You may however get bonus marks for timing the murmur to be in systole (between S1 and S2) or diastole(between S2 and S1). Medical professional will confirm murmur and decide about further management. It is however useful to seek for signs of heart failure i.e. rapid breathing, rapid heart rate, enlarged liver etc which will need urgent attention.

Children can frequently have innocent murmurs which are not due to underlying structural abnormalities. Innocent murmur can be due to fever, severe illness etc however it is difficult to differentiate it from structural defects of heart. It is therefore important to get referral to a paediatrician.

The structural heart defects in children are grouped under common umbrella term "Congenital heart disease " and if it is associate with mixing of pure to impure blood it is called cyanotic congenital heart disease. These babies are blue or dusky and need urgent attention.

Cyanosis is a term indicating poor oxygen supply to the tissues. The oxygen saturation levels that can be tested by saturation monitor, are low (normally 95% or above). The cyanosis **present as bluish lips, tongue and hands, and** can be due to severe respiratory disease, however that baby will have respiratory distress or sternal recessions.

Cyanotic heart disease that may present at 6-8 weeks baby check include transposition of great arteries, abnormal venous return from lungs to right side of heart instead of left and Fallot's Tetrology defect.

There is another group of congenital heart diseases where there is structural defect of heart but there is no mixing of pure and impure blood. These are called "acyanotic heart disease". These are more likely to be seen in health visitor or nurse practice as compared to cyanotic ones which will present to GP or hospital.

Common acyanotic heart diseases are ventricular septal defect, atrial septal defect, patent ductus , coarctation of aorta, pulmonary stenosis, aortic stenosis etc. Ventricular septal defect (VSD) is due to hole in ventricular septum that separates two bottom pumping chambers of heart. As a result there is shunting of blood from left to right ventricle and the flow changes produce a murmur at left lower sternal edge. The typical murmur is long systolic murmur and may cover whole systole. Since the pressure on right side of heart is high at birth but gradually reduce to come to normal around 6 weeks age allowing lot of shunting of blood, babies can go into heart failure.

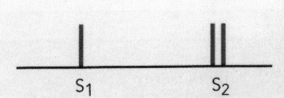

First and (physiologically) split second sound

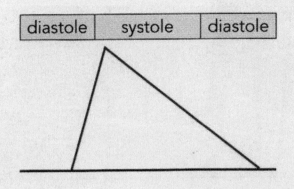

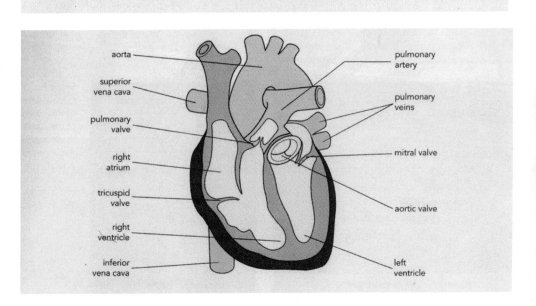

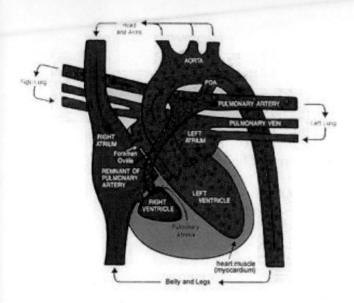

Checking Femoral pulses - Place the tip of your index finger or thumb in the groins, starting midpoint of groin crease that's where the femoral artery ought to be. Slowly adjust the position of your finger tips until you localize the pulse. This is one of the difficult aspects of the baby check, so take your time and be patient! Assess volume – an absent or weak pulse may suggest a coarctation of the aorta. If you are in doubt, ask other professionals and arrange to measure blood pressures on all 4 extremities.

Congenital heart diseases

Congenital cardiac disease occurs in 7-8 per 1000 live births.
- ➢ Most congenital defects are well tolerated in utero and it is only after birth that the impact of the abnormality becomes apparent
- ➢ These may be a part of syndromes, for example:
  - ○ Down's syndrome: AVSD, VSD, ASD
  - ○ Turner's syndrome: coarctation
  - ○ Trisomy 18 / 13: multiple abnormalities

- ➢ Or may be due to drug intake in pregnancy: phenytoin, lithium, warfarin
- ➢ Or infection in pregnancy like Rubella: PDA, VSD, coarctation of the aorta
- ➢ Or maternal systemic disease like SLE: causes heart block , diabetes: causes increased incidence of structural heart disease and hypertrophic cardiomyopathy

Ask History

- ➢ Family history - known congenital problems, affected sibs
- ➢ Perinatal history - cyanosis

- ➢ Feeding - shortness of breath during feeds
- ➢ Poor Weight gain
- ➢ Sweating - especially where cold and clammy
- ➢ Breathing difficulties -tachypnoea
- ➢ Central Cyanosis

Presentation can be in form of first detection of a heart murmur or there can be symptoms
- ➢ Central cyanosis(bluish colour of body)
- ➢ Failure to thrive
- ➢ Poor feeding
- ➢ Symptoms and signs of congestive heart failure
  - o Poor feeding, during which the infant becomes tired
  - o Weight gain which may exceed 30 grams per day, despite the poor feeding
  - o Tachypnoea
  - o Tachycardia with gallop rhythm
  - o Hyperactive precordium
  - o Fine Crackles on auscultation
  - o Hepatomegaly

Pansystolic Systolic Murmurs
- - Ventricular septal defect with a left to right shunt:
- - The murmur is maximal at the left lower sternal edge, and may be loudest when the defect is small
- - 15 -20%
- - Large defects can cause CHF

- - **Inspection**

- o Comfortable
- o Nutrition
- o Cyanosis
- o Pallor
- o Dysmorphism
- o Respiratory Rate and dyspnoea
- o Recessions
- o Sweaty
- - **Palpation**
- - Peripheral Pulses- Presence or absence, Rate, Volume, Differential volumes
- - Precordium   -Hyperactive? ,Thrills
- - **Auscultation**
- - Ejection systolic murmurs
- - ASD (Upper left sternal edge ULSE) Usually isolated defect .5% -10% CHF occurs rarely

- Pulmonary stenosis(ULSE) 8-10% Fatigability, exercise intolerance
- Aortic stenosis (URSE)3-5% Fatigability ,exercise intolerence
- Continuous Murmurs

- PDA
- Machinery murmur
- Upper left sternal edge
- Newborns can go into CHF with PDA

Cardiac murmurs (auscultation sites)
Aortic area
–Right second intercostal space close to the sternum
–Aortic valvular stenosis
Pulmonary area:
–Left second intercostal space close to the sternum
–ASD, Pulmonary stenosis, Coarctation of aorta, PDA
Tricuspid area:
–Inferior left sternal margin
–VSD ,Vibratory Innocent Murmur
Mitral area:
–At position of apex beat
–Mitral regurgitation,Innocent murmur

Summary
➢ History is very important
➢ Pick up cyanosis and consider causes
➢ Examination of CVS can be difficult in a baby
➢ Any sound other than first and second sound can be abnormal
➢ Site where murmur is best heard can be useful
➢ Important to feel for femoral pulses in all babies

It may be tricky for health visitors or nurse practitioners to initially get into concept of auscultation and listening to heart or breath sounds. It is however not difficult after practice and your job is only to screen out normal from abnormal sounds. You do not need to classify the heart sounds or murmurs. Refer to GP or other professional who will make further assessment and decision for referral to specialist.

Meanwhile suggest 3 things you could do to increase your confidence in auscultation of heart and breath sounds?

....

....

....

Respiratory system

Breath sounds –normal and abnormal

Breath sounds are due to air going in and out of lungs, and are hence inspiratory and expiratory. It can be heard by putting stethoscope over chest.

To be able to distinguish between types of abnormal breath sounds and their location, it is important to understand normal respiration and its effect on airway noises that make up breath sounds. Normal breath sounds are bronchovesicular in nature. They are loud pipe-like sounds in the large airways, and softer blowing-like sounds in the small airways. Normal breath sounds are loudest during inspiration and softest during expiration. The inspiratory phase is shorter with faster airflow. Although abnormal sounds may be louder during inspiration, they may be difficult to distinguish due to their short duration.

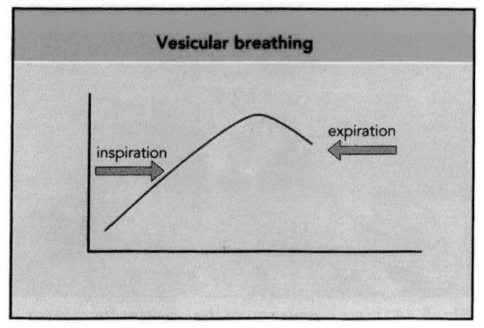

Respiratory Cycle

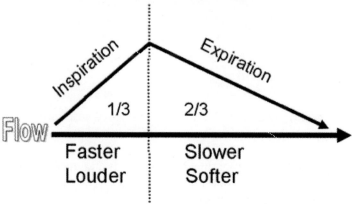

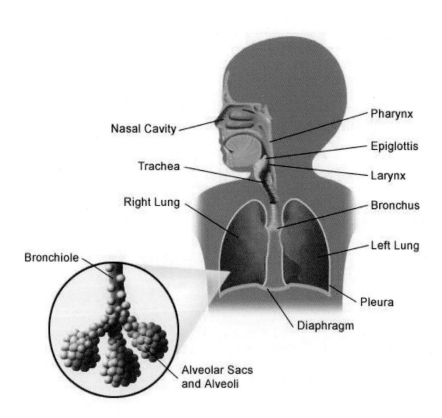

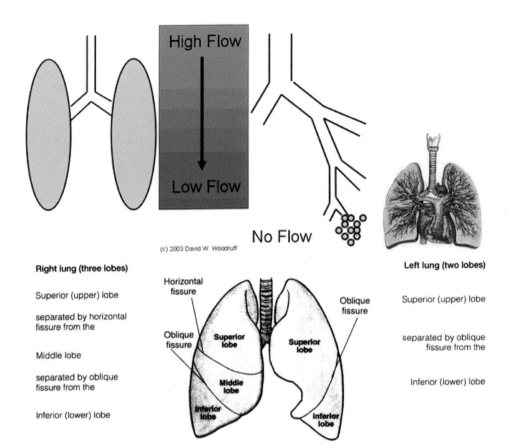

(c) 2003 David W. Woodruff

Right lung (three lobes)

Superior (upper) lobe

separated by horizontal fissure from the

Middle lobe

separated by oblique fissure from the

Inferior (lower) lobe

Left lung (two lobes)

Superior (upper) lobe

separated by oblique fissure from the

Inferior (lower) lobe

Flow is greatest in the trachea and diminishes in the distal lung fields, until it reaches the alveoli, where there is no flow. Breath sounds are loudest over areas with greater flow, and distal pathology may be communicated to these areas. Therefore, auscultation over the trachea may reveal pathology there or communicated from distal regions of the lung.

<u>Wheezing:</u> musical, whistling sound
Usually more pronounced during expiration
From narrowed airways
Bronchoconstriction
Secretions

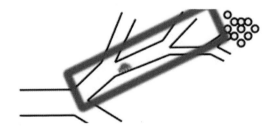

<u>Rales: crackling sound</u>
Heard at the end of inspiration
From collapsed or waterlogged alveoli
Fine: beginning of fluid buildup / or atelectasis
Coarse: greater volume of fluid buildup

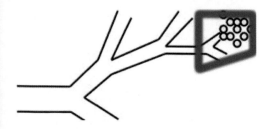

Bronchiolitis

Bronchiolitis is an infection of the lower respiratory tract that usually affects infants. There is swelling in the smaller airways or bronchioles of the lung, which causes obstruction of air in the smaller airways. It mostly occurs in winter and spring. common age group is 2 to 6 months.

The most common cause of bronchiolitis is a virus, most frequently the respiratory syncytial virus (RSV). However, many other viruses have been involved, including: parainfluenza virus, adenovirus, rhinovirus

Initially, the virus causes an infection in the upper respiratory tract, and then spreads downward into the lower tract. The virus causes inflammation and even death of the cells inside the respiratory tract. This leads to obstruction of airflow in and out of the child's lungs.

The following are the most common symptoms of bronchiolitis. However, each child may experience symptoms differently. Symptoms may include:
common cold symptoms, including:

- ➢ runny nose
- ➢ congestion
- ➢ fever
- ➢ cough (the cough may become more severe as the condition progresses)
- ➢ changes in breathing patterns (the child may be breathing fast or hard; you may hear wheezing, or a high-pitched sound)
- ➢ decreased appetite (infants may not eat well)
- ➢ irritability

➢ vomiting

Bronchiolitis is usually diagnosed solely on the history and physical examination of the child. Some times X-ray or blood tests are done. Nasopharyngeal swab - for respiratory syncytial virus (RSV) and other respiratory viruses are used for confirmation.

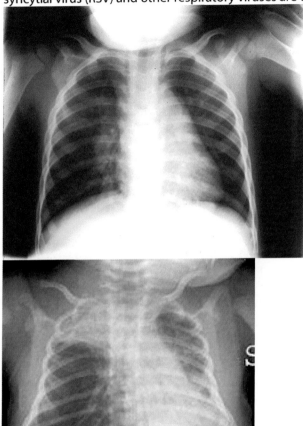

There is no specific treatment for bronchiolitis. Oxygen and nasogastric feeding is given if needed. The rest of treatment is supportive.

Most cases are mild and can be treated at home. Because there is no cure for the disease, the goal of treatment is supportive of the symptoms. Antibiotics are ineffective in the treatment of bronchiolitis. An injection may be given in high risk babies to help decrease the chances of getting respiratory syncytial virus (RSV), which is the most common cause of bronchiolitis. The medication is called Palivizumab (Synagis). Babies in the higher risk category include those who were born prematurely, are less than 6 weeks old, have congenital heart disease, suffer from chronic lung conditions (such as bronchopulmonary dysplasia and cystic fibrosis) or who have compromised immune systems. Other factors that can put infants in a higher risk category are crowded living conditions, exposure to cigarette smoke, attendance in daycare, presence of older siblings in the home and not being breastfed.

Module 12 –Gastro-intestinal system and abdomen

Examination of abdomen

Examination of abdomen and Gastrointestinal system is important as infants at this age suffer from variety of conditions like colic, gastro-oesophagel reflux etc.

Inspection - Look for– distension, symmetry of shape and breathing movement of abdomen.(babies are abdominal breathers). A scaphoid abdomen is seen in diaphragmatic hernia. Umbilicus - note presence/absence of redness, discharge, and odour are signs of infection and may need antibiotic or further work-up. There may be umbilical granuloma or discharge.

Palpation - Use a fairly flat hand, altering the orientation of your fingers so as to get the best possible sensitivity. If the baby is screaming - use the intervals when the baby must inhale to quickly "snatch" a feel. The liver is occasionally palpable - approach the right coastal margin from below with your flat fingers pointing towards the head and dip your fingers up-down to sense the edge, then change the direction of your hand so that your index finger is parallel to the costal margin, keeping some pressure on while letting your hand/index fingers glide carefully from the right iliac fossa towards the costal margin. This way you will occasionally feel the edge of the liver impinging on your index finger. The spleen is not normally palpable, use the tips of your fingers and start your palpation a few cm below the left costal margin, moving/ pushing up towards the lateral part of the costal margin.

The kidneys - are also not normally palpable, but may be felt in skinny/dystrophic infants. Use the tips of your fingers to squeeze down to either side of the umbilicus and then move upwards. Congenital tumors are rare, but important to discover. Use both your fingers tips and your flat hand to palpate all aspects of the abdomen.

Auscultation – It may be omitted unless there are signs/symptoms suggesting an abdominal problem.

Gastro-oesophageal reflux

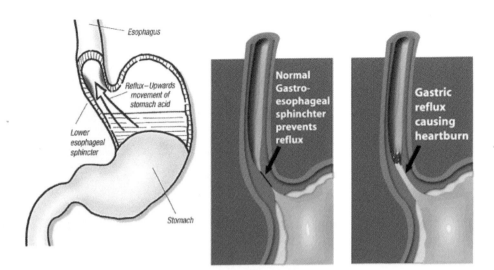

In contrary to our common belief, quite a number of babies also suffer from Baby acid reflux disease , also called Gastro Oesophageal Reflux Disease (GORD). It is most commonly seen in case of babies less than 1 years of age and more frequent during the 3-4 months of life. The symptoms of baby acid reflux is that he will be constantly crying after each feed. There will be belching and pain over the upper abdomen.

Baby acid reflux may cause vomiting of the freshly taken diet, coughing or in most severe cases difficulty in respiration.

Babies who suffer from acid reflux disease must be burped adequately after each feed, this includes all the breast-fed and the bottle-fed babies.
Medication prescribed include Gaviscon, domperidone, ranitidine etc (to neutralize the formed acid). There may be need to change the diet habit of the baby.

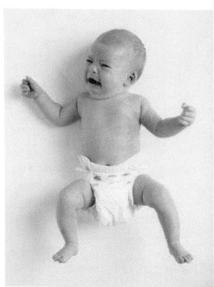
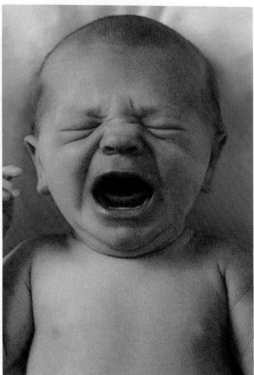

It is not uncommon for newborn babies to go through periods when they appear abnormally irritable or seemingly cry for no reason. However, if you suspect your baby is suffering from colic, you may look for the following symptoms:

➤ cries vigorously for long periods, despite efforts to console
➤ symptoms occur around the same time each day or night, often after meal times, and usually ending as abruptly as they began
➤ shows signs of gas discomfort and abdominal bloating
➤ has a hard, distended stomach, with knees pulled to the chest, clenched fists, flailing arms and legs, and an arched back
➤ experiences frequent sleeplessness, irritability and fussiness

In most cases, colic is the worst pain a baby has thus experienced. It is usually manifested as an acute abdominal pain with intense spasmodic cramping, but since colicky babies cannot describe exactly what distresses them, it is hard for parents to know the precise cause of their distress. Infantile colic is most common in the first few weeks to four months of an infant's life; rarely does it endure past six months of age. Pediatricians often use the "Rule of Three" to diagnose colic: "A baby that cries for three or more hours per day, at least three times per week, within a three month period". Wess, et al., "Paroxysmas fussing in infancy." Pediatrics 1984:74:998. About 25 percent of babies worldwide meet the official "Rule of Threes" criteria for medical diagnosis of colic.

Distension- Children have slightly bulging tummy in first couple of months and it is not too difficult to distinguish when it becomes distended and tight . generally there are other symptoms like vomiting, feed refusal, constipation etc to suggest some bowel pathology and perhaps obstruction. See advice of another medical professional in such situations. Remember Bowel obstruction is an emergency and need to be seen by a doctor as soon as possible.

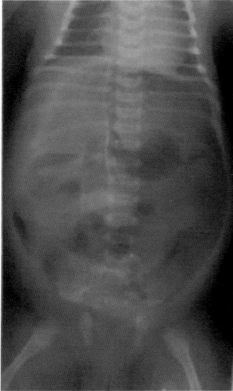

The person doing baby check needs to know about
•Normal anatomy
•Inguinal hernia
•Hydrocele
•Undescended testis
•Testicular torsion
•Ambiguous genitalia

Genitals examination

In Boys

Note the presence of testicles or delayed descent. If you can't feel the testicle, place your index finger higher up in the groin and "milk" your way towards the scrotum, "catching" the testicle between the index finger and thumb of your other hand. Undescended testicles are not unusual (3-4% of term boys), and should be followed up for their descent , surgical referral is generally not demanded till 6-12 months.

Occasionally hydrocele of the testes will be present in term boys. Most of these will disappear during the 1st year of life. Hernia however need an urgent referral in view of risk of obstruction.

Inspect the shaft of the penis to rule out urinary hole in unusual position , i.e. under the surface or over the surface of penis rather than tip - hypo-/epispadias. If such anomalies are present a paediatric surgeon should be consulted. Circumcision is contraindicated in boys with such anomalies, as foreskin will be needed in plastic repair.

Inspect for patency and location of anus and ascertain that the baby pass stools from that opening. The anal opening should be centrally located in the skin "star" formed by the sphincter muscle.

In Girls
The labia majora will cover minora. Check patency of introitus. Occasionally whitish or even blood-tinged secretions will be seen. Unless accompanied by bad smell or other signs of possible infection, such secretions may be normal.

Testis and surrounding structures

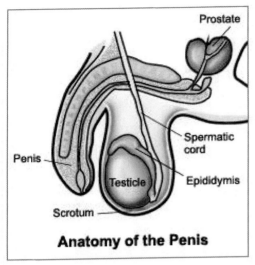

Anatomy of the Penis

Hernia/ hydrocele development

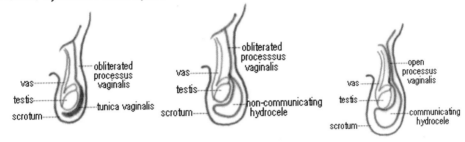

Inguinal hernia

A hernia is described as a protrusion of the contents of abdominal cavity into sac. Commonest hernia is into groin and is called inguinal hernia. A hernia may have piece of bowel into it and may become obstructed. This may cause risk to life and hence all cases of inguinal hernia must be referred to a paediatric surgeon.

An inguinal hernia usually presents itself as a lump in the groin area. The lump may disappear on lying flat, or may be pushed back, only to reappear when coughing or straining. It can cause discomfort (or pain), which often worsens when lifting a heavy object, and tends to increase in size, with time. Occasionally, the hernia can become stuck, and very painful ("strangulated"), in which case urgent surgery might be necessary.

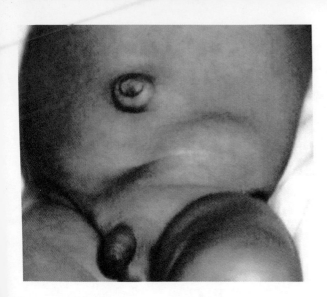

Inguinal hernias

As a male foetus grows and matures during pregnancy, the testicles develop in the abdomen and then move down into the scrotum through an area called the inguinal canal. Shortly after the baby is born, the inguinal canal closes, preventing the testicles from moving back into the abdomen. If this area does not close off completely, a loop of intestine can move into the inguinal canal through the weakened area of the lower abdominal wall, causing a hernia.

Although girls do not have testicles, they do have an inguinal canal, so they can develop hernias in this area as well. It is the commonest surgical condition encountered in childhood . 2.5% of children require an operation for an inguinal hernia. Incidence is increased in premature and low birth weight infants. Male: female ratio is 9:1 . 5% new born male have an inguinal hernia , 70% are right sided , 25% are left sided, 5% are bilateral . 99% are indirect hernias in infancy i.e. they travel same path as testis. 30% present within the first year of life. 15% present with obstruction and 75% of obstructed hernias present less than one year of age .

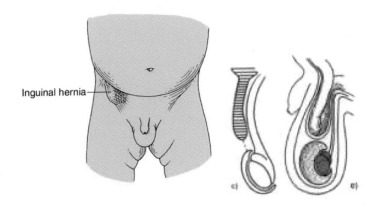

Clinical features of Inguinal hernia

These usually presents with intermittent groin lump. It may come as case of swelling of scrotum or testis. In girls the lump is in the upper part of the labia majora . Hernias can be difficult to detect in a quiet child .Increases in size with straining or crying .May result into Irreducible hernias/strangulation.Initial management should be with reduction by taxis .Required gentle pressure usually without sedation .Forcible reduction under general anaesthesia is contraindicated .If remains irreducible should be operated on within 24 hours, urgent referral needed .If intestinal obstruction present preoperative resuscitation is essential

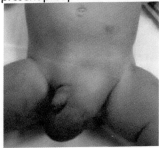

Management

Less than one year old should be operated on as urgent elective basis.
Older than one year surgery is less urgent . It can often be performed as a day case procedure.
Inguinal herniotomy is performed. The wound is closed and the testis pulled back into the scrotum . 20% children develop a contralateral hernia
Controversial as to whether contralateral exploration should be performed.

Hydrocoele

Hydrocoeles are due to fluid accumulation, are commonly present at birth, but may appear in infancy. They present as a scrotal swelling and may be confused with an inguinal hernia. They are due to persistence of the processus vaginalis (a peritoneal projection that accompanies the testicle in its descent into the scrotum). Fluid in the hydrocoele may remain in communication with the peritoneal cavity, so the hydrocoele can change in size. It is important to differentiate them from inguinal herniae (although the two can co-exist). However, there are many causes of inguinal swellings and abnormalities.

In hydrocoele the upper margins can be defined and these are trans-illuminant. The swellings are not tender, and are irreducible.

Fluid accumulates between the two membranes that cover the testicles and one or both testicles may be swollen. Hydrocele swelling gradually increases over a period of weeks or months and is usually painless. There is no impulse on coughing as it is not connected to abdominal cavity if there is no hernia.

Treatment is surgery and the referral to paediatric surgeon is done non-urgent as compared to urgent referral for inguinal hernia (that one may undergo obstruction and strangulation with risk of necrosis of bowel).

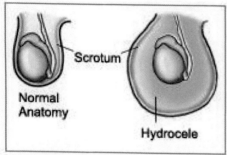
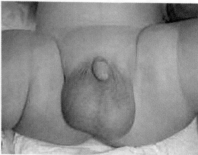

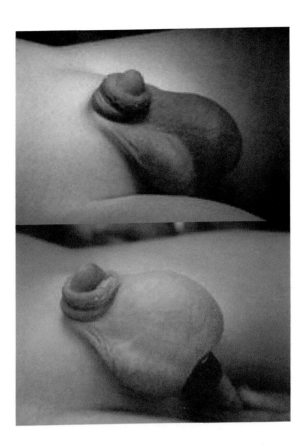

Hypospadias

When the opening of the urinary passage is not on the tip of penis and is rather on lower surface penis (urethra in foetal life develops by folding of skin on under-surface of penis). This results from incomplete fusion of genital folds and glandular urethra . It is on many occasions replaced distal fibrous chordee. The deformity consists of malpositioned meatus, chordee and abnormal foreskin. If any degree of hypospadias is present circumcision is contraindicated .

It affects approximately 1 in 500 boys. 70% are glandular or coronal , 10% are penile, 20% are scrotal . Perineal hypospadias is associated with intersex and anorectal anomalies

Surgical management is required unless urinary meatus is just on undersurface of glans and covered by prepuce to allow normal functioning. The main purpose of surgery is to improve urinary stream and to allow a normal sexual intercourse in future. Surgery is usually performed between 2 and 4 years of age. Glandular hypospadias requires a glandular meatotomy. Coronal hypospadias requires a meatal advancement and glanduloplasty (MAGPI operation). Proximal hypospadias without a chordee can be treated by a skin flap advancement. If chordee present it should be excised and an island flap urethroplasty performed

Cryptorchidism

If testis is not in normal position it is called cryptorchidism (testis in abnormal position). It may be a Normal' testis i.e. retractile testis that has gone up from scrotum or Abnormal' testis that has never been seen low in scrotum and can not be manipulated to that position.

Testicular descent

Testis is normally formed in abdomen in foetal life near kidney. It undergoes intra-abdominal descent up to 28 weeks of intrauterine development. It is normally found in inguinal canal from 28-32 weeks onwards and should be expected to be found in scrotum from 30 weeks onwards. In full-term infants incidence of cryptorchidism is 6% and by three months incidence has fallen to 2% . A high incidence of cryptorchidism is seen in premature infants.

Undescended testis is less common than perceived. In 80% of patients referred with cryptorchidism the testis is palpable. 90% of impalpable testes are either high in inguinal canal or abdomen. True absence of testis is rare and is due to either primary agenesis or neonatal torsion. Cryptorchidism increases the risk of testicular tumours by x10 and 10% of patients with testicular tumours give a history of testicular maldescent . Cryptorchidism increases risk of infertility. Of patients with cryptorchidism - 30% have oligospermia and 10% azospermia

Undescended testis

Undescended testis is generally found in normal path of descent. It is usually found in inguinal canal or abdomen. Maldescended testis has exited via the superficial inguinal ring but is now in an ectopic position. Usual sites are the femoral triangle or perineum

Empty maldeveloped scrotum indicated that testis has never descent.

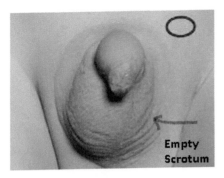

Management of the undescended testis

If testis palpable in inguinal canal or high in scrotum patient requires orchidopexy. It should be performed during second year of life. Usually performed via 'groin and scrotum' incision to place it back in position and fix)called orchidopexy). Early orchidopexy may improve fertility. No evidence that it reduces risk of malignancy but allows early identification. If testis is impalpable laparoscopy is best means of identifying intra-abdominal testis, vas and vessels.

Testicular Torsion

Testicular swelling that is painful indicates either there is inflammation or torsion of testis. Torsion happens due to twisting of spermatic cord and risk is cutting off blood supply leading to necrosis of testis.

Umbilical granuloma

It is not uncommon and is seen as red granulomatous tissue on umbilicus. It is painless and not infected. It is due to failure of epitheliasation which should happen to make it look like a normal skin. Chemical cauterisation with silver nitrate application cause the granulomatous tissue to die and thus healing with epithelial skin.

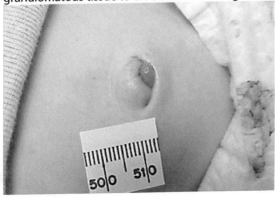

Umbilical hernia

Umbilical hernias are common in infancy, occurring in as many as 1 in 6 children. They are due to incomplete closure of the ring of muscle around the umbilical ring through which the umbilical vessels enter the fetus.

They are more common in preterm infants, in children with Down Syndrome, and children with hypothyroidism. It is important to differentiate umbilical hernias from small omphalocoeles.

Most umbilical hernias close spontaneously within 3-5 years. Large hernias are less likely to close than small hernias and, as compared to inguinal hernias, incarceration is very rare. It is commonly suggested that treatments such as taping a coin to the hernia to keep it in, or strapping it, will promote resolution. Whilst unlikely to do any harm, these strategies do not have any beneficial effect. If the hernia is still present at the age of 3, referral to a paediatric surgeon may be indicated.

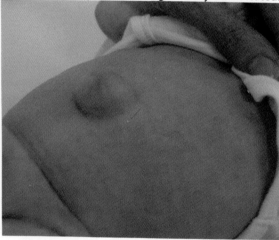

Examination of hip

The most important part of the musculoskeletal examination at 6-8 weeks baby check is the evaluation of hips and lower extremities. The hips are examined for the possibility of dislocation. Congenital dislocation of the hip involves a lack of development of the acetabulum and femur. Inspect the contours of the legs while the child is lying supine. The presence of asymmetrical skin folds on the medial aspect of the thigh is suggestive of a proximally dislocated femur.

Early diagnosing of dysplasia and hip joint dislocation

History of dislocation in first degree relative and breech delivery are strongly associated with increased risk.

Symptoms :

1. Restriction of abduction in the hip joint. Degree of the restriction in the hip joint abduction depends on the form of hip joint disorder. So with dysplasia the abduction is less restricted and with dislocation it is more severe. To find this out you should put the baby on his back, bend its legs in the hip and knee joints at right angles and put his legs to the sides. If the movement is restricted (it is more noticeable with one-sided pathology) you should clarify the reason for restriction You should keep in your memory the fact that with age the ability to abduct the hips to 90 o decreases and at the age of 9 months makes only 50 o .

Figure showing restriction of abduction in the hip joint with one-sided hip dislocation in newly-born infants.

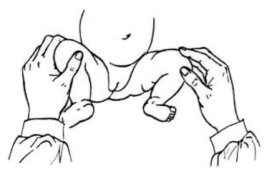

2. Sliding symptom or the symptom of a «click» is called Marks's and Ortolani symptom. When the baby's legs are abducted you can sense reset of dislocation with a distinctive click and knock.

The click symptom is positive during the first three months of life (Ortolani).

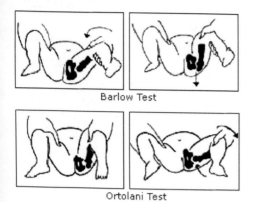

Barlow Test

Ortolani Test

Barlow Test— Fold both legs at the knees and grasp the folded legs between the lengths of your index finger and thumb. Place your middle finger so that it parallels the femur on the dorsal side, and put the tip of your middle finger on the trochanter. This test is positive when the hips are held in 90 degrees of flexion and pressure is applied over the lesser trochanter while adducting the hip, forcing the femoral head out of the acetabulum. When the pressure is released, the dislocatable hip usually returns into the acetabulum. The idea behind the Barlow maneuver is to diagnose lax or subluxated hip joints.

I find that it helps me to perform this maneuver correctly if I imagine the femoral head riding on the edge of the hip socket. I then visualize pushing the femoral head backwards so that subluxated becomes luxated, such than when I follow with the Ortolani maneuver, I will feel the 'clunk' described above.

An infant with a positive Barlow test needs confirmation and referral.

Ortolani Test—Fold both legs at the knees and grasp the folded legs between the lengths of your index finger and thumb. Place your middle finger so that it parallels the femur on the dorsal side, and put the tip of your middle finger on the trochanter. Flex the hips to right angles relative to the pelvis and trunk and then abduct. As you approach maximal abduction, use the tips of your middle fingers to lift the proximal end of the femur forwards. A positive sign will consist of a feeling of a 'clunk' as the femoral head slips into the socket. This is known as the Ortolani maneuver.
I find that it helps me to do the exam correctly if I maintain a mental image of the femoral head being dislocated posteriorly (which is usually the case), and my task is to use my fingertips to lift the head into the socket.

It is better if each hip is tested independently while the opposite side of the pelvis is stabilized.

3. Asymmetry of hip, buttock and popliteal region folds. Asymmetry of hip folds as well as their unequal number testify to the existence of dysplasia or dislocation. Very often asymmetry of buttock folds indicate one-sided or bilateral hip dislocation. However this symptom is not an absolute one as asymmetry of folds, especially hip fold can be observed in health babies as well.

4. Shortening of the lower extremity. It can be easily seen when you put a baby on his back with the legs bent in knee joints at right angles. You can compare the length according to the position of ankles and heels when the legs straightened.

Fig showing Detection of hip/thigh shortening with one-sided hip dislocation.

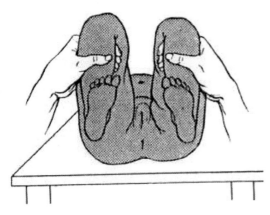

5. External [outward] rotation of lower extremity. This symptom is most easily observed in the one side when compared with the healthy leg. External [outward] rotation is especially visible when the baby is asleep and the mother can pay attention to it.

6. In case of congenital hip dislocation greater trochanter on the side of the dislocation is more massive and is projecting under surrounding tissues and stands out higher.

7. To diagnose the pathology in case of dysplasia or hip joint dislocation suspicion-ultrasound or X-ray examination may be required.

Developmental dysplasia of hip

Developmental dysplasia of the hip is a congenital (present at birth) condition of the hip joint. It occurs once in every 1,000 live births. The hip joint is created as a ball and socket joint. In DDH, the hip socket may be shallow, letting the "ball" of the long leg bone, also known as the femoral head, slip in and out of the socket. The "ball" may move partially or completely out of the hip socket.

Familial predisposition

The greatest incidence of DDH occurs in first-born females with a history of a close relative with the condition.

Hip dysplasia is considered a "multifactorial trait." Multifactorial inheritance means that many factors are involved in causing a birth defect. The factors are usually both genetic and environmental.

Often, one gender (either male or female) is affected more frequently than the other in multifactorial traits. There appears to be a different "threshold of expression," which means that one gender is more likely to show the problem than the other gender. For example, hip dysplasia is nine times more common in females than males.

One of the environmental influences thought to contribute to hip dysplasia is the baby's response to the mother's hormones during pregnancy. A tight uterus that prevents fetal movement or a breech delivery may also cause hip dysplasia. The left hip is involved more frequently than the right due to intrauterine positioning.

Risk factors for developmental dysplasia of the hip (DDH)

First-born babies are at higher risk since the uterus is small and there is limited room for the baby to move; therefore affecting the development of the hip. Other risk factors may include the following:

- family history of developmental dysplasia of the hip, or very flexible ligaments

- position of the baby in the uterus, especially with breech presentations

- associations with other orthopaedic problems that include metatarsus adductus, clubfoot deformity, congenital conditions, and other syndromes

The following are the most common symptoms of DDH. However, each baby may experience symptoms differently. Symptoms may include:

the leg may appear shorter on the side of the dislocated hip
the leg on the side of the dislocated hip may turn outward
the folds in the skin of the thigh or buttocks may appear uneven
the space between the legs may look wider than normal

A baby with developmental dysplasia of the hip may have a hip that is partially or completely dislocated, meaning the ball of the femur slips partially or completely out of the hip socket.

Developmental dysplasia of the hip is sometimes noted at birth. The pediatrician screens newborn babies in the hospital for this hip problem before they go home.

However, DDH may not be discovered until later evaluations. At 6-8 weeks baby check it is important to pick it up.

When clinically suspected diagnostic confirmation is usually done by ultrasound (sonography.) – Commonly used diagnostic tool for DDH. It is a imaging technique which uses high-frequency sound waves and a computer to create images of blood vessels, tissues, and organs. Ultrasound produce picture of acetabulum cavity of hip

joingt and head of femur and their relative position.

X-ray is generally used in older infants.

Treatment- The goal of treatment is to put the femoral head back into the socket of the hip so that the hip can develop normally.

The Pavlik harness is used on babies up to 6 months of age to hold the hip in place, while allowing the legs to move a little. The harness is put on by your baby's physician and is usually worn full time for at least six weeks, then part-time (12 hours per day) for six weeks. Your baby is seen frequently during this time so that the harness may be checked for proper fit and to examine the hip. At the end of this treatment, x-rays (or an ultrasound) are used to check hip placement. The hip may be successfully treated with the Pavlik harness, but sometimes, it may continue to be partially or completely dislocated.
traction and casting

If the hip continues to be partially or completely dislocated, traction, casting, or surgery may be required. Traction is the application of a force to stretch certain parts of the body in a specific direction. Traction consists of pulleys, strings, weights, and a metal frame attached over or on the bed. The purpose of traction is to stretch the soft tissues around the hip and to allow the femoral head to move back into the hip socket. Traction is most often used for approximately 10 to 14 days. Traction can either be set up at home or in the hospital, depending upon your baby's physician, hospital, and the availability of the resources.

If the other methods are not successful, or if DDH is diagnosed after the age of 18 months, surgery may be required to put the hip back into place manually, also known as a "closed reduction." If successful, a special cast (called a spica cast) is put on the baby to hold the hip in place.

There is some debate as to the effectiveness of ultrasound as screening test for the at-risk groups.

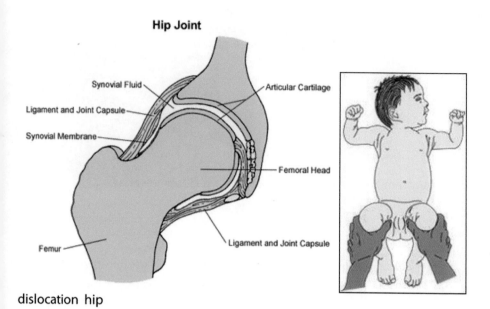

Hip Joint

Synovial Fluid

Ligament and Joint Capsule

Synovial Membrane

Articular Cartilage

Femoral Head

Femur

Ligament and Joint Capsule

dislocation hip

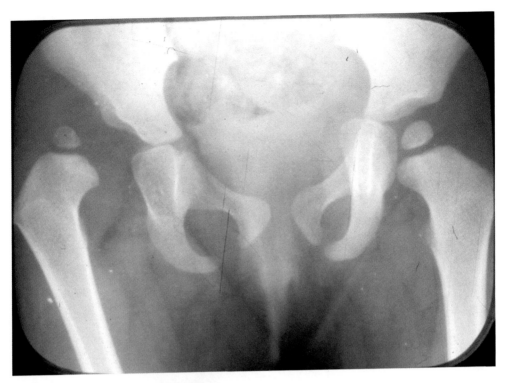

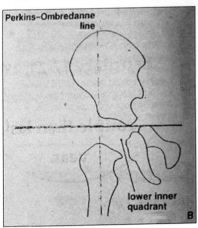

Perkins–Ombredanne line

lower inner quadrant

B

The Perkins-Ombredanne line is drawn perpendicular to the Y-line, through the most lateral edge of the ossified acetabular cartilage, which actually corresponds to the anteroinferior iliac spine in normal newborns and infants, the medial aspect of the femoral neck or the ossified capital femoral epiphysis falls in the lower inner quadrant. The appearance of either of these structures in the lower outer or upper outer quadrant indicates subluxation or dislocation of the hip.

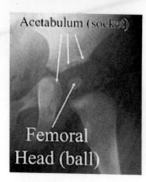

Acetabulum (socket)

Femoral
Head (ball)

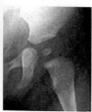 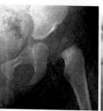 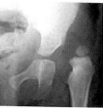

dislocation left and sublaxation right

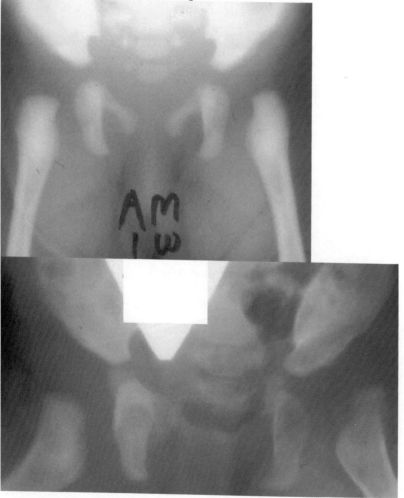

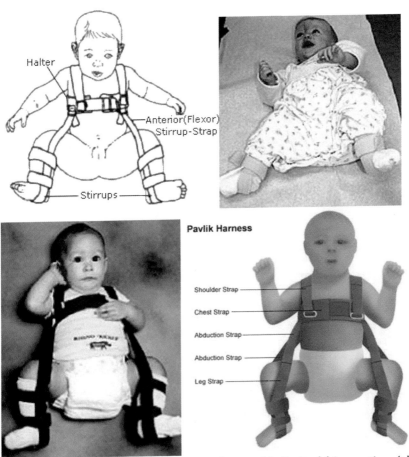

Pavlik Harness

The Pavlik harness can be used in infants with limited hip motion (abduction) and ultrasound or X-ray abnormalities. The Pavlik harness is generally used for 2-3 months for 23 hours a day and may be followed by a short period of nap and nighttime wear.

bilateral dislocation, more on right

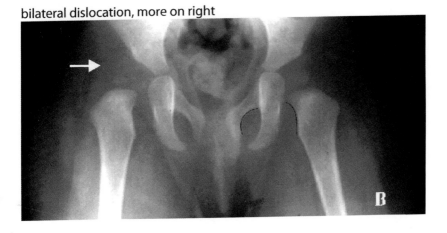

While newborn screening for DDH allows for early detection of this hip condition, starting treatment immediately after birth may be successful. Many babies respond to the Pavlik harness, traction, and/or casting. Additional surgeries may be necessary since the hip dislocation can reoccur as the child grows and develops. If left untreated, the baby may have differences in leg length, and may limp.

Eczema

A diagnosis of eczema can be tricky because it's easily confused with a number of other skin conditions and infants are especially prone to rashes. Be sure to provide a detailed description of when and how you discovered the rash and whether or not your baby was experiencing any other symptoms at the time.

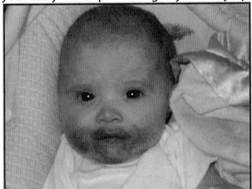 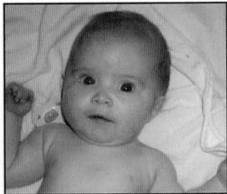

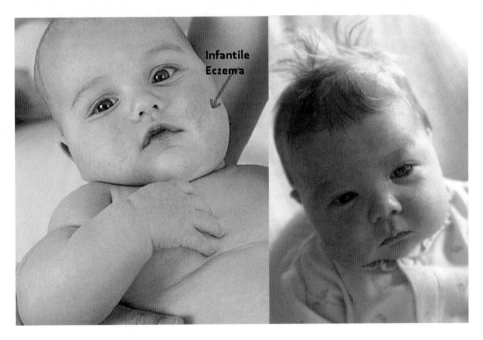

Infantile Eczema

Mongolian spot = It may be noticed as an ill defined blue-blackish area of skin over the lumbosacral area in 90% of Native American, black and Asian infants.

It is due to the presence of pigmented cells in the deeper layers of the skin. Become less noticeable as pigment in overlying cells becomes more prominent and disappear in early childhood.

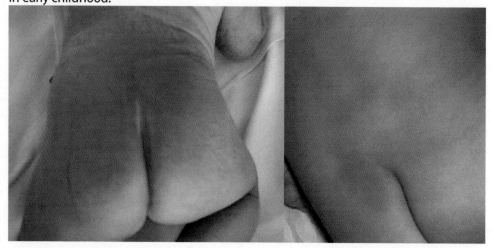

Acrocyanosis: Hands and feet "blue" at birth and remain so for several days. May recur throughout early infancy when baby is cold. A blue colour or hands is acceptable in cold weather but a blue colour or tongue is indicative of central cyanosis and need urgent referral.

Capillary malformations: Flat vascular birthmarks can be divided into two types: those that are orange or light red (salmon patch) and those that are dark red or bluish-red (port-wine stain). The salmon patch is a light red macule found over the nape of the neck, upper eyelids and glabella. 50% of infants have such lesions over their necks. Eyelid lesions fade completely within 3-6 months; those on the neck fade somewhat but usually persist into adult life. Port-wine stains are dark red or purple macules appearing anywhere on the body. A bilateral facial port-wine stain or one covering the entire half of the face may be a clue to *Sturge-Weber syndrome*. Most infants with smaller, unilateral facial port-wine stains do not have Sturge-Weber syndrome. Similarly, a port-wine stain over an extremity may be associated with hypertrophy of the soft tissue and bone of that extremity (Klippel-Trenaunay syndrome).

Hemangioma

Haemangioma is a red, rubbery nodule with a roughened surface. The lesion is often not present at birth but is represented by a permanent blanched area on the skin that is supplanted at age 2-4 weeks by red nodules. Hemangiomas may be superficial, deep or mixed. Histologically, these are benign tumors of capillary endothelial cells. 50% resolve spontaneously by age 5 years, 70 % by age 7 years, and 90% by age 9 years; leaving redundant skin, hypopigmentation, and telangiectasia.

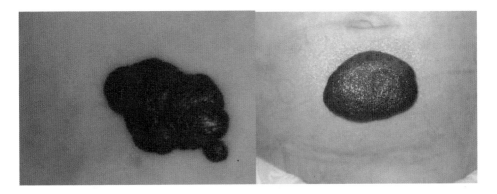

Lymphatic Malformations: Lymphatic malformations may be superficial or deep. Superficial lymphatic malformations present as fluid-filled vesicles often described as looking like frog spawn. Deep lymphatic malformations are rubbery, skin-colored nodules occurring in the parotid area or on the tongue. They often result in grotesque enlargement of soft tissues.

Café au lait spots (pigmented spots)

These are dark brown spots that need to be watched and may be associated with genetic disease like neurofibromatosis.

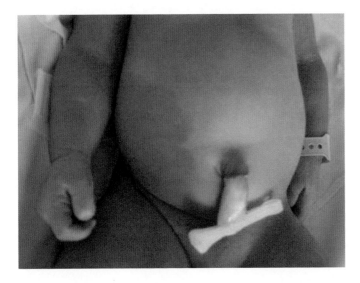

Nappy rash is a common problem for neonates within the first few months of life. Whilst the exact aetiology of nappy rash is not clear, it is felt to be due to moisture in the nappy environment and from irritation from urine and stool. Many infants will be affected by superinfection with Candida albicans.

Typically in Candidal nappy rash, there is erythema in the perineal region, with satellite lesions which may coalesce. There is often an appearance of scale. In the images to the left from the same baby, satellite lesions are seen. Note that there are some lesions close to the umbilicus and extending around the flank. Swabs were positive for Candida.

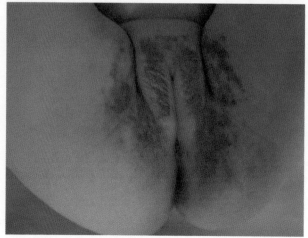

Treatment primarily involves the use of a topical agent such as nystatin or miconazole. There should be liberal use of barrier creams, and soiled and wet nappies should be changed promptly. Oral nystatin may be used in conjunction with topical treatment, although this may not improve resolution. Occasionally, in severe cases, a mild topical steroid may be needed.

Conditions that need to be considered in the differential diagnosis include psoriasis, contact or irritant dermatitis, and zinc deficiency.

Seborrhoeic dermatitis

Seborrhoeic dermatitis primarily affects the scalp and intertriginous areas. It is most common in the first 6 weeks of life, but can occur in children up to 12 months of age. Involvement of the scalp is frequently termed "cradle cap", and manifests as greasy, yellow plaques on the scalp. Other commonly affected areas include the forehead and eyebrows (as in the photo to the left), nasolabial folds, and external ears. Involvement of skin creases, such as the nappy area, can lead to secondary Candidal infection and maceration.

The aetiology is unknown. Treatment includes the use of a mild tar shampoo, oatmeal baths, and avoidance of soaps. Occasionally, a mild topical steroid may be indicated.

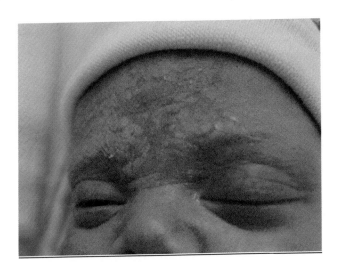

Staphylococcal infections

Staphylococcal scalded skin syndrome is an acute epidermolysis caused by a staphylococcal toxin. Newborns and children are most susceptible. Symptoms are widespread bullae with epidermal sloughing. Diagnosis is based on examination and very rarely skin biopsy.

The condition is aggressive and treatment with intravenous Penicillinase-resistant antistaphylococcal antibiotics must be started immediately. Prognosis is excellent with timely treatment. It can be confused as burn.

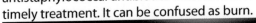

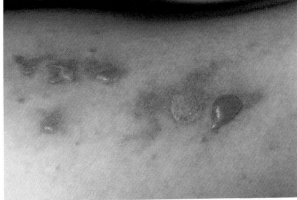

Bruise and child protection concerns should always be kept in mind

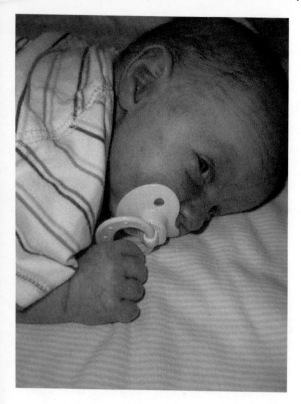

Communication to parents about examination

Health visitors and practice nurses are quite good in conversation to parents however additional skill and confidence may be needed to feel comfortable talking about the organs or systems they were not very familiar with. It may also need skills in breaking bad news if there is any abnormality detected.

The health visitors and practice nurses also need to have skills in communicating to the other health professionals regarding their new skills and the challenges resulting from newly acquired skills. Normally you have good access to the general practitioners, however it will be useful to be assertive and discuss the issues that you are not comfortable with or if you are suspicious of any abnormality in baby check.

Since the system varies from place to place and the nature of general practice also very, some health visitors and nurse practitioners have found it useful to set aside some time to discuss cases with GPs. It is a skill to be non-confrontational but be assertive for expressing the view about findings.

Module 17 – Assessment Quiz

The assessment quiz is available online, please check the voucher in book or ask your trainer for entry code.

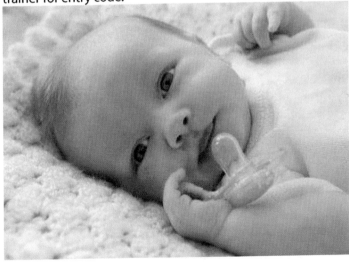

What did you learn?

Knowledge...

....

....

....

....

Examination skills..

....

....

....

....

Communication skills ....

....

....

....

....

Observation skills...

....

....

....

....

Other...

....

....

....

....

....

....

....

....

....

Practical experience sheets

Please write reflective notes. Gibbs' reflective cycle can be really useful in making you think through all the phases of an experience or activity. This course is not one stop shop for learning but starting a process of continued development in knowledge and skills. You will have enough knowledge and skills to do the baby checks but you will encounter many new things just like you find in life experience. Many of our candidates have seen what they haven't seen before or have dealt with a situation or challenge in an interesting way. They have learnt much more briefly writing on these sheets, particularly Evaluation phase. It gave more confidence for future baby checks. As a practitioner it is easy to be too conscious of the things that didn't go well. Don't be too hard on yourself! The Evaluation phase makes you think about the positive as well as areas for improvement.

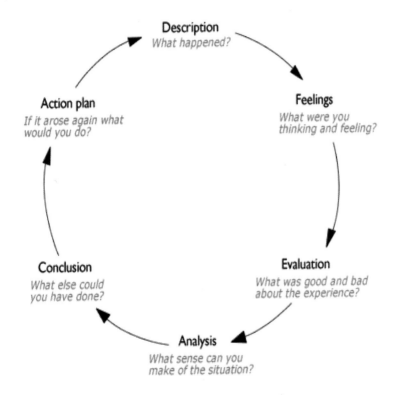

The examination of the 6-8 week old Child

Learning Outcomes and Competency Log

Competency	Observed	Supervised	Unsupervised
1. Assess family history in relation to child's age and condition	1 2 3 Comments	1 2 3 Comments	1 2 3 Comments
2. Critically appraise pregnancy, perinatal problems and type of delivery and the effects that these might have on the child including prematurity	1 2 3 Comments	1 2 3 Comments	1 2 3 Comments
3. Demonstrate the ability to undertake a full physical examination on a child aged 6 to 8 weeks in order to detect any abnormalities.	1 2 3 Comments	1 2 3 Comments	1 2 3 Comments
4. Demonstrate proficiency in the use of a stethoscope in detecting normal heart and respiratory sounds and any other abnormalities.	1 2 3 Comments	1 2 3 Comments	1 2 3 Comments
5. Demonstrate proficiency in the detraction of cyanosis, respiratory distress and heart murmurs.	1 2 3 Comments	1 2 3 Comments	1 2 3 Comments
6. Demonstrate competence in the identification of dysmorphic features and congenital abnormalities	1 2 3 Comments	1 2 3 Comments	1 2 3 Comments
7. Demonstrate competence in the identification of squint, nystagmus and abnormal pupils.	1 2 3 Comments	1 2 3 Comments	1 2 3 Comments

Competency	Observed	Supervised	Unsupervised
8. Demonstrate competence in the use of the ophthalmoscope to detect abnormalities and red reflex	1 2 3 Comments	1 2 3 Comments	1 2 3 Comments
9. Demonstrate ability identify any abnormalities of the mouth and palate	1 2 3 Comments	1 2 3 Comments	1 2 3 Comments
10. Palpate the abdomen and detect any palpable mass/organ	1 2 3 Comments	1 2 3 Comments	1 2 3 Comments
11. Identify a range of communication skills in order to deal with a critical situation i.e. breaking bad news, difficult parents/sibling	1 2 3 Comments	1 2 3 Comments	1 2 3 Comments
12. Provide rationales for referral to agreed agencies	1 2 3 Comments	1 2 3 Comments	1 2 3 Comments
13. Demonstrate competence in the examination of the hips i.e. Ortolani and Barlow Method	1 2 3 Comments	1 2 3 Comments	1 2 3 Comments

Competency	Observed	Supervised	Unsupervised
14. Assess child's alertness and responsiveness appropriate for 6-8 weeks	1 2 3 Comments	1 2 3 Comments	1 2 3 Comments
15. Assess posture and tone of upper and lower limbs to detect abnormality	1 2 3 Comments	1 2 3 Comments	1 2 3 Comments
16. Assess head control in ventral suspension and prone.	1 2 3 Comments	1 2 3 Comments	1 2 3 Comments
17. Demonstrate the ability to interpret abnormalities in results of screening tests i.e. Guthrie, Neonatal Hearing test	1 2 3 Comments	1 2 3 Comments	1 2 3 Comments
18. Demonstrate competence in the examination of the fontanelles and identification of abnormalities.	1 2 3 Comments	1 2 3 Comments	1 2 3 Comments
19. Assess skin for abnormalities i.e. birth marks, bruises, rashes and jaundice	1 2 3 Comments	1 2 3 Comments	1 2 3 Comments
20. Assess normal appearance of genitalia in males and females and recognise any deviations. Detect hernia.	1 2 3 Comments	1 2 3 Comments	1 2 3 Comments

Competency	Observed	Supervised	Unsupervised
21. Assess normal appearance of genitalia in males and females and recognise any deviations. Detect hernia.	1 2 3 Comments	1 2 3 Comments	1 2 3 Comments

Health Visitors 6-8 weeks baby check course - Review

Why did you do the course?

What did you gain from it?

What is the value of health visitor doing 6-8 weeks check as compared to GP?

Have you been able to do some baby checks with supervisor?

Have you practiced 6-8 baby check on your own?

Does it give you a sense of special satisfaction?

How do you view it doing in practical life?

What do envisage the hurdles in HV doing 6-8 weeks checks?

Do you feel health visitors as a group can overcome the problems?

Any other comment ....